THE NEW PEDIATRICS

SOCIAL PROBLEMS AND SOCIAL ISSUES

An Aldine de Gruyter Series of Texts and Monographs

SERIES EDITOR

Joel Best

Southern Illinois University at Carbondale

Joel Best (*editor*), **Images of Issues: Typifying Contemporary Social Problems** (Second Edition)

Joel Best (*editor*), **Troubling Children: Studies of Children and Social Problems**

Anne E. Figert, **Women and the Ownership of PMS: The Structuring of a Psychiatric Disorder**

James A. Holstein, **Court-Ordered Insanity: Interpretive Practice and Involuntary Commitment**

James A. Holstein and Gale Miller (*editors*), **Reconsidering Social Constructionism: Debates in Social Problems Theory**

Gale Miller and James A. Holstein (*editors*), **Constructionist Controversies: Issues in Social Problem Theory**

Philip Jenkins, **Intimate Enemies: Moral Panics in Contemporary Great Britain**

Philip Jenkins, **Using Murder: The Social Construction of Serial Homicide**

Valerie Jenness, **Making It Work: The Prostitutes' Rights Movement in Perspective**

Stuart A. Kirk and Herb Kutchins, **The Selling of *DSM*: The Rhetoric of Science in Psychiatry**

John Lofland, **Social Movement Organizations: Guide to Research on Insurgent Realities**

Bruce Luske, **Mirrors of Madness: Patrolling the Psychic Border**

Leslie Margolin, **Goodness Personified: The Emergence of Gifted Children**

Donna Maurer and Jeffrey Sobal (*editors*), **Eating Agendas: Food and Nutrition as Social Problems**

Dorothy Pawluch, **The New Pediatrics: A Profession in Transition**

Erdwin H. Pfuhl and Stuart Henry, **The Deviance Process** (Third Edition)

William B. Sanders, **Gangbangs and Drivebys: Grounded Culture and Juvenile Gang Violence**

Theodore Sasson, **Crime Talk: How Citizens Construct a Social Problem**

Wilbur J. Scott, **The Politics of Readjustment: Vietnam Veterans since the War**

Wilbur J. Scott and Sandra Carson Stanley (*editors*), **Gays and Lesbians in the Military: Issues, Concerns, and Contrasts**

Malcolm Spector and John I. Kitsuse, **Constructing Social Problems**

Robert A. Stallings, **Promoting Risk: Constructing the Earthquake Threat**

Frank J. Weed, **Certainty of Justice: Reform in the Crime Victim Movement**

THE NEW PEDIATRICS
A Profession in Transition

DOROTHY PAWLUCH

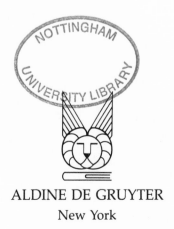

ALDINE DE GRUYTER
New York

About the Author

Dorothy Pawluch is Assistant Professor in the Department of Sociology at McMaster University in Hamilton, Canada. She received her Ph.D. from McGill University. In addition to professions and social problems, Dr. Pawluch's interests include alternative health care.

ALDINE DE GRUYTER
A division of Walter de Gruyter, Inc.
200 Saw Mill River Rd
Hawthorne, New York 10532

This publication is printed on acid free paper ∞

Library of Congress Cataloging-in-Publication Data
Pawluch, Dorothy, 1953–
    The new pediatrics : a profession in transition / Dorothy Pawluch.
        p.   cm. — (Social problems and social issues)
    Includes bibliographical references and index.
    ISBN 0-202-30534-1 (cloth : alk. paper)
    1. Pediatrics—Social aspects—United States.   2. Pediatrics—Practice—United States.   3. Pediatrics—United States—Philosophy.
    I. Title.   II. Series.
    RJ47.7.P38   1996
    618.92—dc20   96-1029
                                                               CIP

Manufactured in the United States of America

10 9 8 7 6 5 4 3 2 1

Contents

Foreword

Dorothy Pawluch, Associate Professor of Sociology at McMaster University in Hamilton Ontario, already well known in her discipline for her signally thoughtful critique of theories of social problems, here presents a full-length empirical study of the medical specialty of pediatrics. The results are rich in insight, thoughtful and surprising. Professor Pawluch recalls the finest period of the "old" University of Chicago tradition of Hughes, Blumer, Becker and Strauss, in which the researcher plunged into a social world, learned its language and history, its secrets, its hopes and fears, and then produced an ethnographic and interpretive account that made contributions to a whole range of specialties within sociology. In this book, students of social movements will find a new case study in the emergence of pediatrics in the nineteenth century. Students of the professions will appreciate the care that Pawluch lavishes on the transformation of pediatrics, a "profession in process," and in the discussion of the emergence of new "segments" within pediatrics and their complicated interrelations. Her discussion of the human impact of transforming technologies on the individual practitioners—the care providers, not the care recipients—is virtually unique in our field. Students of deviance and the sociology of social problems will find grist for their mill in her discussion of "the new pediatrics" and the extension of medical solutions to "behavior problems" of all kinds. Finally, all those disciplines concerned with the role of the child in society must pause to think about the inner world of the profession that for over a century has argued that children and their problems, medical and otherwise, are different and also claimed that it, better than anyone else, understands these problems.

However, because Professor Pawluch writes in such an engaging and nontechnical style, this book can be read in another way. Each chapter paints a vivid picture of the doctor and the child-patient at different periods. These pictures are not, however, simply portraits of medical heroes. Each one has an element that is in some way disturbing. These pictures invite us to play the children's game "What is wrong with this picture?" Let us then imagine a series of pictures of a child being examined by a doctor, like the cover of this book.

In one picture, the child is extremely ill. Doctor A, however, knows nothing about the diseases of children. There is no such knowledge. The child dies. Looking at the face of the mother, we see resignation mixed with sadness. She knows that many children do not survive. Of her six children, she hopes that maybe four will grow up to become adults.

In another picture, the child is extremely ill, but Doctor B seems fairly confident. Doctor B has seen many cases similar to this one. The doctor prescribes a complicated form of treatment, which now (some 70 years later) has been completely forgotten and abandoned. The child survives. Doctor B is a heroic figure to the child's parents. They only have two children and both are extremely precious to them. Some people might say, however, that the city's much improved water supply, better refrigeration and preparation of food, and other improvements in public health saved this child.

In a third picture, Doctor C explains to the mother how to disguise the foul taste of the latest miracle drug, some gigantic pill or evil–tasting syrup. On the way out of the office, a nurse hands the mother a pamphlet explaining the importance of getting a series of shots to inoculate against the traditional list of childhood killers. Doctor C sometimes thinks that pediatric medical practice has now been reduced to writing out prescriptions for one new drug after another. If you look carefully, you may see that the doctor is vaguely restless, and yes, a little bored.

In a later picture, the child is abundantly healthy. She comes in for her routine checkups, but very little ever seems to be the matter with her. In fact, when a really sick child comes in, Doctor D gets nervous. Doctor D no longer has much experience with serious illness. Doctor D refers the really sick child to Doctor E, a specialist at an internationally famous teaching hospital. The boredom that had so subtly infiltrated the demeanor of Doctor C in the previous picture is abundantly clear in this one. On the corner of Doctor D's desk you may see applications for residencies in gerontology!

Here is an odd picture. How did this one get in here? Perhaps it was meant for a different book? But no. The "child" appears to be 14 years old, perhaps even older. He is having problems in school and perhaps that is the school guidance counselor standing in the corner. I see the next patient sitting in the waiting room. Her problem seems to be traumatic feelings about her pimples and acne. Neither of these patients is "ill." But does Doctor F look bored? Not at all. Trained as a pediatrician, Doctor F now has a practice limited to "Behavioral adjustment disorders of adolescents." A bunch of nurse practitioners seem to have taken over Doctor F's former "well-baby" practice.

Well, these are just some of the images brought to mind by Dorothy Pawluch's fascinating chronicle of the rise of pediatrics, its several crises, and its sometimes surprising transformations. She brings to her story the training of a professional sociologist, the patience and skills of a historian, and a fiercely independent spirit that allows her to distance herself from the self-congratulatory back slapping of both the medical biographers and also of the critics of modern medicine.

This book will interest anyone who wonders how the accelerating pace of medical innovations affects not only the patient, but the doctors—their hopes, fears, dreams, pocketbooks, plans, and careers. It will help people understand how the current array of primary care institutions for children emerged out of a peculiar set of institutions that developed when children were much sicker and no one knew how to cure them. Professor Pawluch provides context to understand the recent aggressive expansion of medical treatments for behavior problems, and she identifies the process through which one or several types of primary health care professionals will survive the competition to treat the next generation of children. Although her home discipline is sociology, all disciplines and persons interested in the evolution and future of health care will profit from following the absorbing story so well told in these pages.

Malcolm Spector Ph.D., JD
New York

Acknowledgments

The story about pediatrics that I tell in this book had its origins in a dissertation, narrower in focus, begun at McGill University well over a decade ago. The debts that I have incurred in transforming that initial analysis into what appears in these pages are enormous. As I was finishing the final chapters of the manuscript, Richard Koffler, who as executive editor at Aldine de Gruyter was well aware of the numerous stumbling blocks I had run into along the way, sent me a wonderfully encouraging letter that ended: "All the propitiatory divinities have been smiling on your work, Dorothy." I readily, and gratefully, acknowledge the role that Divine Providence played. But God has worked His wondrous ways through the many caring and generous individuals that He has placed along my path. I hope that those I have neglected to mention by name here will forgive me.

First and foremost I thank Malcolm Spector. Malcolm was there as an advisor when this work started, as a friend when it ended and at so many critical points in between. The influence of Malcolm's thinking and writing will be apparent to those who know his work. But in so many more ways, big and small, Malcolm guided me through this study. It is no exaggeration to say that without him the book would never have been completed. Beyond his contributions to this book, Malcolm has taught me, through word and deed, what it means to be a good sociologist. He has counseled me with wisdom and kindness through critical career decisions. He is a valued mentor and friend. I feel honoured and deeply privileged to have had the opportunity to study and work with him.

At Aldine de Gruyter I thank Richard Koffler for disproving everything I had ever been told about what it was like to deal with publishers. He has been patient, gracious and supportive, and has extended himself well beyond the call of duty. I am grateful as well for his dogged determination to see this thing through. To Arlene Perazzini I extend thanks for her attention to the production details.

To Joel Best, advisory editor of Aldine de Gruyter's Social Problems and Social Issues series, I am grateful for exceedingly helpful comments and for including the book as part of the series. Joseph Schneider's interest in my work has been longstanding. I appreciate the various ways he found to cheer me on over the years.

For their input into the earliest versions of my work on pediatrics and their support while I was at McGill University I am indebted to Prue Rains, Joan Stelling, Jim Robbins, Joseph Lella, Steve Woolgar, Cathy Boyd, Ted Withers, Janice Sager, Irene Lepine, Danielle Champoux and Axel van den Berg. At Concordia University I thank Joseph Smucker and David Howes. My friends and colleagues in Hamilton and at McMaster University have provided me with an environment that has been warm, intellectually stimulating and easy to come back to. I thank Lynne Lohfeld, Jane Aronson, Vivienne Walters, William Shaffir, Richard Brymer, Roy Hornosty, Jack Richardson, Charlene Miall, Eli Teram, Jacqueline Low, Robert Phripp, James Gillett and especially Roy Cain, who has been such a good listener.

Marjorie MacKinnon, Lise Heroux and James Csipak have given me the gift of their friendship—steadfast, nurturing and true.

Towards my family I feel the kind of gratitude that words can scarcely express. My parents, Marie Filomena (Giove) and Theodor, have worked so hard to provide for their children the opportunities and choices they never had. They have always trusted us to make the right choices and their faith in us has been abiding. I hope that this book, in some small way, makes them feel that their faith was not misplaced. I thank Catherine for baby-sitting services rendered, for being my "rock" and for so much more. I thank Tony, Sonia, Andrew and Adam for their love and many kindnesses. I thank George Zaralis for giving me the time and space to write, and for motivating me to finish. Finally, I am grateful to my precious Alexandra for so cheerfully making the sacrifices required of her. I dedicate this book to her and to all children, with a mother's dream for a life lived fully and fulfilled. After all, though we may not always agree on how to achieve it, isn't that ultimately what any of us really want for our children?

Chapter 1

Introduction

CHANGING DEFINITIONS OF PEDIATRICS

Over the last several decades the practice of pediatrics has changed radically—so much so that pediatricians often describe their specialty today as the "new pediatrics," or refer to the problems they treat as the "new morbidity" in pediatrics. What makes the new pediatrics "new" is its shift away from the physical problems of children, which once dominated pediatrics, to problems of a nonphysical nature. While in the past pediatricians were primarily concerned with treating and preventing life threatening infectious diseases, those practising the specialty in most of North America today deal with problems such as temper tantrums, sibling rivalry, bedwetting, eating and sleeping disorders, fears and phobias, shyness, nightmares, thumb-sucking, nervous tics, nailbiting, glue-sniffing, stealing, fire-setting, running away, using obscene language, overdependent relationships with parents, school difficulties, reactions to chronic illness, adoption, and traumatic experiences such as child abuse.

This is only a partial list of the wide range of difficulties that now fall under the pediatric purview. The "new pediatrics" oversees not only children's physical growth and development, but their emotional, psychological, social, and even, as some pediatricians have interpreted it, their spiritual well-being. "We must not only be doctors of the body and of the mind," one pediatrician has written, "but doctors of the spirit as well. If we study, learn and apply ourselves to [spiritual healing], if we see every patient visit as an opportunity to prevent [the erosion of values and quality of family life], we will become effective counselors and true healers" (Atkinson, 1985:333).

Another feature of the new pediatrics is its concern with adolescents. Until the 1950s, pediatricians primarily treated children under the age of 12. Today, many pediatricians follow their patients through their teens, and, in some cases, into young adulthood. Adolescent health care has its own distinctive problems: acne, sports injuries, and the gynecological

1

needs of young women. But since adolescence is the healthiest stage in the life cycle in physical terms, providing health care for teenagers really means attending to behavioral and psychosocial concerns such as sexual activity and birth control, gender preference, peer relationships, relations to authority figures, truancy and school drop-outs, as well as drug abuse.

As dramatic as these changes have been for pediatricians, their impact has not been limited to the practitioners of the profession. The new pediatrics is linked to a shift in the way that we as a society think about children, teenagers, and their difficulties. In redefining pediatrics and extending the limits of their professional responsibilities, pediatricians have, in effect, redefined and medicalized many behaviors that they now treat. Behaviors that were once unnamed or unnoticed, those that we once thought we could do nothing about, or that we might have been prepared to overlook or to accept as a normal part of growing up, now evoke concern. Conditions that were once attributed to random variation in character, aptitude, appetite, and energy level, or to "normal" teenage rebelliousness, we now understand within a medical frame of reference as symptoms of an underlying condition. Behaviors that we once punished, are now referred to pediatricians and other doctors or experts. Labels such as "hyperkinesis" or "hyperactivity," "minimal brain dysfunction," "attention deficit disorder," "learning disability," "dyslexia," "psychosocial dysfunction," or "behavioral dysfunction" have replaced labels such as "naughty," "mischievous," "rambunctious," "lazy," "shy," "stupid," "wild," and "delinquent." Deviance has become disease and medical treatment has replaced discipline as the appropriate way to deal with many troublesome behaviors.

Many people, especially parents, have welcomed and even pushed for greater involvement of pediatricians in children's lives with its promise of more effective management, if not a total "cure," for their nonphysical difficulties and a less troubled, disrupted, and conflict-ridden passage for them into adulthood. But there have been critics as well, charging that the medicalization of childhood misbehaviors is no more than a massive and insidious program of child control and a justification for using medical techniques, including drug therapy, to bring into line those behaviors in children that adults find objectionable, annoying, or bothersome. For example, Shrag and Divoky (1975), two journalists specializing in educational issues, have argued that medical labels and treatment for childhood deviance became popular with the advent of the children's rights movement of the 1960s and the general liberalization of attitudes that made overtly coercive means of maintaining order unpopular, if not illegal. Disease labels met "the political and social necessities of an age searching desperately for an explanation to [the classic problem of deviance] and for a scientific replacement for the golden rule and the hickory stick" (Shrag and Divoky, 1975:48). These disease labels continue to be popular, especially among the middle class, they insist, because they are less stigmatizing than moral labels like "delinquent," they absolve parents of blame for their children's misbehaviors, and allow them to maintain their belief that white, affluent, middle-class families cannot produce children who cannot learn and do not behave. Breggin and Breggin (1994) describe Ritalin, an amphetamine prescribed for hyperkinesis, as a way of regimenting and restraining spirited kids. Others (Castel, Castel, and Lovell, 1982) suggest that medical labels for childhood misbehaviors are often thin disguises for the difficulties that children experience in adjusting to specific, social, family, or scholastic situations. Commenting on the near pandemic proportions of diagnosed learning disabilities, Castel et al. (1982:202), write:

> It is common knowledge that the American educational system is particularly insufficient in some areas. Perhaps this is why cause and effect are often reversed, and pupils are made responsible for the poor performance of the school system—a conspicuous example of blaming the victim.

This book is not about the legitimacy of the new pediatrics, the "true" nature of childhood problems, or whether pediatricians are justified in having absorbed behavioral problems into their professional mandate. These questions are discussed only because they have been raised and debated by pediatricians themselves as the specialty has moved into new areas of care. Nor is this book about why views of many childhood behaviors and issues have changed in recent decades—there are so many forces that have contributed to the shift.

My focus is rather on why pediatricians have been willing to assume responsibility for the problematic behaviors of children and teenagers, and to provide services they never previously considered part of their specialty. I focus specifically on pediatricians because they share what Eliot Freidson (1970a:127) has called the "moral authority" of the medical profession. Doctors, Freidson (1970a) has argued, by virtue of their acknowledged technical expertise, have the power and official mandate to decide what will be regarded as disease and who will be regarded as sick. They act as "final arbiters" over matters of health and illness. In practising a medical specialty devoted to children, pediatricians have been in a position to arbitrate questions dealing with the health and illness of children. By incorporating problematic behaviors into the boundaries of proper pediatric care and providing services in these areas, pediatricians have implicitly legitimized and given official approval to the medical definitions of children's nonphysical problems. If we are more likely to see children's behavior as health care concerns, it is largely because pediatricians have endorsed this view. Their role in how so much of childhood has become medicalized, then, has been pivotal.

What accounts for the rise of the new pediatrics? In this book I demonstrate that the new pediatrics was the outcome of a series of crises that shook the specialty after 1950. Over the first half of the twentieth century, the infectious diseases of childhood came under control and the health of children improved. Pediatrics began to experience difficulties. The rates of infant and childhood death (mortality) and illness (morbidity) fell. This did not directly affect the university-based professors of pediatrics who continued to teach and do research on the physical problems of children. Nor did the change affect the small group of consulting pediatric subspecialists who concentrated on studying and treating the serious, though relatively rare, medical conditions that still struck children. The group hardest hit by the improvements in children's health were the thousands of general pediatricians in private, primary care practice.

The problem was not that these pediatricians had fewer patients to treat. On the contrary, the growing popularity of pediatricians as doctors of choice for children and the postwar baby boom combined to create an overwhelming demand for pediatric services. The problem for primary care pediatricians lay in the kind of medicine they found themselves practising. Their practices increasingly consisted of preventive work— weighing and measuring babies and otherwise supervising the normal growth and development of their young patients—and the treatment of minor illnesses that were easily handled or disappeared on their own without any treatment at all. The growing frustration and boredom with such practice generated a crisis of purpose for the specialty. The crisis, which pediatricians themselves referred to as the "dissatisfied (or disgruntled) pediatrician syndrome" (Pless, 1974:227; Vandersall, 1963) was a pervasive sense of malaise among primary care pediatricians who doubted whether their specialized, disease-oriented skills were serving any real purpose in child health care. It was in the context of the dissatisfied pediatrician syndrome that some within the specialty began to suggest the primary care pediatrics could be revitalized if pediatricians addressed themselves to children's unmet needs, particularly those that were not strictly medical. Pediatricians were encouraged to be creative in their exploration of new areas of care.

Key segments within the profession resisted the expansion of pediatrics into nonphysical areas. But the specialty's ambitions in these new areas were fortified during the 1970s when another crisis hit—a supply crisis. Pediatricians found themselves competing for a dwindling child population with new groups of health care practitioners eager to provide their services to children, pediatric nurse practitioners, and the budding specialty of family practice. This supply crisis pushed the specialty further toward the new pediatrics. The new pediatrics became more than just a way to make the practice of primary care pediatrics rewarding and fulfilling. It was now the linchpin in pediatricians' assertions that they were the professional group best equipped to deal with children's total health care concerns.

Pediatricians, then, were not seeking to gain a greater measure of control over children's lives. Indeed, as this book will show, they have, somewhat reluctantly, absorbed the new pediatrics into their practices. What they were seeking to do was to preserve a place for themselves in primary child health care at a time when their role in the area was threatened. By redefining what proper pediatric care involves to include the new pediatrics, they hoped to secure a future for themselves as primary care practitioners. But in the process, they altered fundamentally our view of children, their problems, and their lives.

The developments in pediatrics that this book describes have been limited largely to North America. Children in the third world have not benefited to the same degree as North American children from advances in scientific and medical knowledge. Over 97% of children in developed countries reach the age of 5, while in developing countries, 20–25% of all children die before reaching their fifth birthday (UNICEF, 1990:29). An estimated 13 million children under the age of 5 die annually in developing countries; the corresponding figure for the developed world is in the range of 135,000 (UNICEF, 1994:82). Pediatricians in these countries generally treat children under 12 years of age and face conditions similar to those that characterized pediatric practice in North America around the turn of the twentieth century. Infectious and gastrointestinal diseases, aggravated by poverty and malnutrition, are rampant. Pediatricians are not primary health care providers as they are in North America. In Europe, pediatricians are consultants. They have not expanded their practices into behavioral problems to the same extent as their North American counterparts. Rather they concentrate on the treatment of physical disease.

AN OVERVIEW

The book is organized in the following way. While it is customary for studies such as this to begin with a discussion of their theoretical underpinnings and methodological approach, I have decided to reserve these discussions for later. Those who are interested, will find them in the final chapter and in a methodological appendix, both of which are better read as conclusions to the book. Those less interested will be able to read the book to this point without an interruption in the flow of the analysis and without the distraction of abstractions.

Instead, I begin with a chapter that provides the background knowledge about pediatrics needed to understand the crises that are the focal point of my analysis. Chapter 2 presents a necessarily brief and cursory overview of pediatrics as an organized specialty in the United States. It traces the evolution of the specialty from its inception in the late 1800s until the 1950s, when the dissatisfied pediatrician syndrome first surfaced. I describe the circumstances surrounding the emergence of pediatrics and pediatricians' early interest in artificial or bottle feeding. I also describe the developments that eliminated pediatricians' baby feeding role, reduced levels of infant and child mortality and morbidity, and pushed pediatricians ultimately into prevention.

Chapter 3 focuses on the dissatisfied pediatrician syndrome. The chapter begins with a documentation and explanation for the growth in preventive and routine care as a component of pediatric practice. It then continues to examine the impact on practising pediatricians. I look in a detailed way at the long and emotional letters pediatricians wrote via their professional journals to their colleagues, expressing their disaffection and questioning their career choices. I show how some pediatricians responded by suggesting that the specialty needed to find new challenges, while others resisted what they saw as a fundamental and problematic redefinition of the specialty's scope of practice.

In Chapter 4, I trace the emergence of new groups of health care providers interested in children and the supply crisis that their appearance precipitated in pediatrics. What factors gave rise to the creation of pediatric nurse practitioners and the rejuvenation of general medicine in the form of the family practitioners? How did pediatricians react to their appearance and growth? And what impact did they have on the movement to take pediatrics into a new, more comprehensive approach to child health care? These are the central questions addressed in the chapter.

Chapter 5 is about the strategies that those who supported the new pediatrics used to promote their vision of the specialty and to encourage new patterns of practice among primary care pediatricians. I look specifically at three strategies: the formulation of an explicit and forceful rationale to justify new directions for the specialty, the formalization of the new pediatrics as the profession's standard of proper child health care, and the reform of educational programs.

The success of these strategies in institutionalizing the new pediatrics is assessed in Chapter 6, which also deals with pediatrics' future prospects.

In the final chapter I present some concluding observations about the new pediatrics and take up the book's theoretical context. In tracing the new pediatrics, I draw on a theoretical perspective that has gained wide currency in sociology. For some readers, it will be enough to know that the perspective, known as *social constructionism*, stresses the actor's point of view. That explains why my concern, throughout the book, is on why pediatricians felt they needed to expand their professional boundaries rather than on the merits of the new pediatrics. Chapter 7 presents a fuller treatment of social constructionism—what it is about, where it originated, and how it has developed. The chapter also examines the related literature on medicalization, that is, on the production of medical constructions and interpretations. I take a closer look at studies that touch, in one way or another, on medicalization as it has affected children's lives and describe how my analysis fits in with those studies. I also reflect on what the new pediatrics tells us about professions as claimsmakers or constructors of reality.

Finally, a word about the appendix. The appendix provides a description of how the study was prepared, the data used, and what I learned about studying professions. With the hope that these experiences may benefit those interested in doing similar work, I suggest specific research strategies, highlighting in particular the value of the professional literature. I also examine some of the methodological and difficult conceptual concerns that arise when, as a constructionist, one attempts a study of this sort.

Chapter 2

A Brief History of Pediatrics: A Background

INTRODUCTION

Pediatrics had its beginnings as an organized specialty in the United States in the late 1800s when a small group of doctors with a growing interest in studying and treating the diseases of children united to create the first formal pediatric organizations in the country. Initially they called themselves "pediatrists" and their area of interest was called "pediatry" or "pedology" (King, 1993:69). But by the beginning of the 1900s these terms were replaced by "pediatrician" and "pediatrics," probably to prevent confusion with podiatry, a term that refers to the study of diseases of the foot (Cone, 1979:70). Over the next several decades pediatrics grew into one of the most popular and thriving specialties in medicine. In this chapter I cover the key moments and central organizational milestones in that development.

The facts are more than merely historically interesting. The crises that gripped the specialty after the 1950s and culminated eventually in the new pediatrics were the consequence of a process that began much earlier. They were rooted in how pediatrics evolved as a primary care specialty and in the distinctive shape of pediatric practices in North America, where the majority of practitioners worked in private, primary care practices rather than in consulting positions. It was the specialty's stake in primary care and its determination to preserve its presence at that level of care that fueled the drive toward the new pediatrics. In this chapter I explain how pediatrics acquired that stake.

The chapter begins with the circumstances surrounding the rise of organized pediatrics at the end of the last century, the rapid growth of the specialty through the first several decades of this century, its early interest in the illnesses of children, especially those connected with artificial or bottle feeding, and the significance of the pediatrician's role as "baby feeder" in the consolidation of pediatrics as a branch of medicine. The next part of the chapter then focuses on how the decline of infectious diseases began to reduce the need for pediatricians' curative skills, entirely eliminated the need for pediatricians' baby feeding work and led gradually to the differentiation of the specialty into segments with contrasting work patterns. While a small number of pediatricians moved into highly specialized areas of care and practiced as subspecialists, others moved into full-time, private, primary care where they supported themselves by providing preventive as well as curative services. That is, in addition to treating sick children, they monitored the growth of healthy children. The inclusion of prevention in pediatricians' work and the move into primary care were the basis of the specialty's continued growth until the 1950s, but it was also the basis of the crises it later faced.

CONTEXT AND EMERGENCE

The health of children when pediatrics came on to the scene as an organized specialty was as bad as it probably ever has been (Rosen, 1975:3–6). The incidence of disease or morbidity and the mortality rates among infants and young children during the late 1800s tell the story. Twenty to forty percent of all infants born alive died during the first year of life. Half of all children died before their fifth birthday. Of the total number of deaths in the population, three out of every four occurred in children under 12 years of age. The greatest killers were infectious diseases such as cholera infantum (summer diarrhea), typhoid fever, dysentery, tuberculosis, diphtheria, pertussis (whooping cough), scarlet fever, influenza, and pneumonia. Nearly half of all deaths due to infectious diseases occurred in infants and children under 5 years of age (Table 2.1). "Human life," as one pediatrician (Lucas, 1927:2) described it, "was cheap."

Despite the desperate plight of children, or perhaps because of it, most people through the nineteenth century reacted to the high rates of mortality and morbidity among infants and young children with an attitude of acquiescence and quiet resignation. They viewed childhood as a perilous prospect and accepted the fact that a high proportion of children would simply never make it to adulthood. Families experienced the death of a child as a dreaded loss. But at the same time they expected at least some of their children to die and would often leave a newborn baby nameless for several months lest they "waste" a favorite name (Ehrenreich and English, 1979:185).

The same attitude of resignation permeated medical ranks. Most doctors were not involved with sick children. They might respond to specific requests for their services, but rarely sought children out as

Table 2.1. The Ten Leading Causes of Death in Childhood: 1850[a]

Children Under 1 Year		Children 1–4 Years	
1.	Croup	1.	Dysentery
2.	Dysentery	2.	Scarlet fever
3.	Convulsions	3.	Croup
4.	Pertussis	4.	Cholera
5.	Pneumonia	5.	Fever
6.	Cholera infantum	6.	Pertussis
7.	Fever	7.	Pneumonia
8.	Cholera	8.	Cephalitis
9.	Tuberculosis	9.	Worms
10.	Scarlet fever	10.	Convulsions

Children 5–9 Years		Children 10–19	
1.	Scarlet fever	1.	Tuberculosis
2.	Cholera	2.	Cholera
3.	Dysentery	3.	Fever
4.	Fever	4.	Typhoid fever
5.	Typhoid fever	5.	Dysentery
6.	Croup	6.	Pneumonia
7.	Dropsy	7.	Dropsy
8.	Cephalitis	8.	Accident
9.	Pneumonia	9.	Cephalitis
10.	Tuberculosis	10.	Scarlet fever

[a] Smillie (1955) has noted that many of the diagnostic categories, such as fever, convulsions, and worms, are not clearly defined. On the basis of his analysis of the records, Smillie concludes that diphtheria, scarlet fever, and intestinal infections (cholera infantum, cholera, dysentery, convulsions, and worms) were leading causes of death in children under five. Tuberculosis was an important cause of death in infants, dropped in importance for the next 15 years, and then became the leading cause of death in the 10–19 age range.

Source: Adapted from Smillie (1955:206).

patients. They regarded the diseases of young children as "too trivial . . . too abrupt, elusive and fatal to warrant the physician's intervention" (Rosenberg, 1983:2). Infancy, like old age, was seen as a time to die (Dye and Smith, 1986:344). Abraham Jacobi, one of the first pediatricians and the recognized "father of American pediatrics," described the prevailing attitude in this way: "the diseases of small children are small things" (Jacobi, 1889a:17). Another of the early pediatricians (Casebeer, 1883) complained about the remarks he often heard from colleagues:

We have often been pained by the remarks dropped from the lips of some physicians . . . such as, "Well, you may give a few drops of paregoric or some catnip tea or most anything of that kind you may find convenient, as we cannot do much for children so young" or "Your mothers or 'old women' can treat young children as well as I or any physician can;" or "I don't like to treat children. It is so unsatisfactory. They cannot tell how they feel and what is the matter with them, and I never can tell what they need." (Casebeer, 1883:327)

Since so few doctors were willing to treat children it was left to parents, grandparents, neighbors, and experienced mothers and midwives in the community to minister to the sick or dying child. Though midwives did not consider the treatment of sick children central to their work, they did what they could when asked.

From the point of view of children, perhaps it was just as well that doctors avoided them. When they did treat sick children, most doctors used anecdotal remedies that were at best ineffective and often fatal (Preston and Haines, 1991:12). Medical historians have described the medical treatment of children as "one of the saddest aspects of nineteenth century practice" (Coulter, 1969:113). Since the infectious diseases that struck so persistently among children were usually characterized by fever and since blood-letting was the accepted treatment for fevers, children were routinely bled. The object was to draw enough blood to induce fainting or to temporarily stop the pulse. When the patient was a child the jugular vein was used because other veins were too hard to find. The jugular vein had the advantage of being easier to locate. But at the same time it made it much harder for doctors to control blood flow, which meant that some young patients eventually bled to death. Another common treatment of the day was the administration of minerals such as mercury, magnesium, lead, iron, copper, zinc, arsenic, and potassium. Though doctors took the diminutive size of children into account in determining dosages, they still used these minerals in massive quantities that often proved lethal. Researching the case of a 1-year-old youngster being treated for violent vomiting, fever, a distended abdomen and diarrhea, one incredulous expert found the prescribed doses of minerals so excessive he consulted the U.S. Bureau of Weights and Standards to see if the measures at the time were comparable to contemporary standards. To his dismay, he found that they were (Gittings, 1928:6). In assessing the impact of these therapies Thomas Rotch (1891:8), another founder of the specialty, had to admit: "It is no exaggeration to state that a large number of sick infants and young children throughout the land are suffering from the vigorous treatment of their zealous medical attendants, rather than from the disease with which they started."

Through the 1800s and the beginning of the 1900s, however, attitudes towards children changed both among the public and within the medical profession (Bremner, 1971:811). Zelizer (1985:26–27), for example, notes that through the nineteenth century there was a new sensitivity about the death of children and a revolution in child mourning. The death of a child became an overwhelming tragedy. "Traditional parental restraint gave way to unabashed outpouring of sorrow" (Zelizer, 1985:25). By the end of the century, the revolution had expanded. Childhood death became more than a family's private grief—it was redefined as an intolerable social loss, a collective, public failure. Equanimity gave way to widespread concern about the conditions of childhood, especially the plight of the urban poor.

The reasons for this shift are still being debated by social scientists. The change in attitude in both North America and Europe has been linked to falling birth rates, which made children less numerous and therefore more valuable (Rosen [1958] 1993; Shryock, 1936), falling mortality rates, which made them safer emotional investments (Aries, 1962; Musgrove, 1964; Stannard, 1977; Stone, 1977), the separation of work and home life brought on by industrialization, which changed the meaning of family relationships and intensified emotional bonds between family members (Dye and Smith, 1986; Laslett, 1978), and the domestication of women, at least, middle-class women (Degler, 1980; Dye and Smith, 1986). Tiffin (1982) suggests that the change had to do with a transformation in the image of children. The child as innately sinful gave way to a more romantic view of children as the purest, most innocent form of human life and, therefore, in need of protection. There is a debate as well about whether those who pressed for reforms for children were motivated by humanitarian impulses (Tiffin, 1982) or by a desire on the part of direct elites to control and dominate the socialization of children, particularly working class and immigrant children, at a time of major social upheaval (Cohen, 1985:273–277; Finkelstein, 1985:112-115; Lasch, 1979; Platt, 1969).

Whatever its source, the new attitude toward children led to intense private and then public activism on their behalf and to what gradually came to be known as the child welfare movement. A host of special services, programs, and institutions were created not only for sick children but for the destitute, neglected, abused, deserted, handicapped, maladjusted, and delinquent. A variety of "child saving" groups and agencies formed including Children's Aid Societies and Societies for the Prevention of Cruelty to Children. Child labor laws, mandatory schooling regulations, and juvenile courts came into existence. Special institutions were established for children including houses of refuge (reformatories), foundling homes or orphanages, infant asylums, dispensaries, and children's hospitals (Zietz, 1959:40–78). It was the establishment of children's hospitals in particular, Halpern (1982; 1988) and others (Jones, 1983; King, 1993:61–68) have argued, that was the most significant spur in the rise of the new specialty. Children's hospitals provided the institutional context within which doctors could begin to develop an interest in the medical problems of children.

The first children's hospital was the Nursery and Child's Hospital founded in New York in 1854. The Children's Hospital of Philadelphia was established in 1855, the Chicago Hospital for Women and Children in 1865, and the Boston Children's Hospital in 1869. Through the 1870s more than a dozen other hospitals for children came into being. Most of these hospitals were small, converted family homes with no more than 20 beds (Golden, 1989). They were funded by private boards of philanthropists and staffed by volunteers. The boards would ask prominent doctors in the community to provide their medical services. Halpern (1988) found that virtually all of the founders of organized pediatrics combined their private general practices with charitable work in such children's hospitals and in other institutions for the young.

These doctors saw first hand the ravages of infectious diseases on young children and became committed to establishing pediatrics as a branch of medicine. This did not mean that they wanted pediatrics recognized as an exclusive area of practice. Like so many other doctors at that time, they were suspicious of complete specialization and did not feel that doctors should be limiting themselvess to any particular aspect of medicine. But they did want children recognized as legitimate objects of medical attention, and the study and treatment of their diseases recognized as legitimate pursuits within medicine. Their common purpose and work patterns gave them an identity that set them apart from other doctors and ultimately combined to create what Halpern (1988:86–87) refers to as "an impulse to organize."

The impulse to organize, Halpern adds, was fueled by another major trend of the late nineteenth century, the move toward specialization in medicine. Specialization was the product of changes in medical thinking about the causes of disease. By the mid-1800s traditional views about the nature of disease had begun to break down and were giving way to a new clinical viewpoint. Diseases were no longer thought of in holistic terms as generalized states of physiological imbalance, but as problems connected to specific organs within the body. The principle of localized pathology or specificity of disease led some doctors to focus on the functioning and malfunctioning of particular organs. At the same time others within medicine were beginning to narrow their interests to the use of particular technologies such as surgery, or to particular treatment techniques such as climatology, which involved using weather conditions to treat respiratory illnesses. Climatology was popular in the late

1800s as a result of its success in the treatment of tuberculosis, but disappeared as more effective treatments were developed.

Gradually these specialists began to organize. They began by creating separate sections within the American Medical Association (AMA), but quickly discovered the resistance among their generalist colleagues within the organization. While voicing a concern about the fragmentation of medicine and its implications for the quality of medical practice, the generalists sensed a potential threat from the specialists. The AMA, therefore, was not the best place for the emerging specialists to pursue their narrower professional interests. They began to form their own groups. The first of these was the American Ophthalmological Society organized in 1864. Over the next two decades other specialty organizations came into existence including the American Otological Society (1867), the American Neurological Association (1875), the American Dermatological Association (1876), the American Gynecological Association (1876), the American Laryngological Association (1879), the American Surgical Association (1880), and the American Climatological Association (1883).

These organizations all preceded the formal organization of pediatrics. But their existence contributed to the rise of pediatrics in several ways. First, they established the principle of specialization within medicine. Second, they gave pediatricians an added incentive to organize themselves. Finally, they provided pediatricians with a model to follow when they did organize.

THE GROWTH OF ORGANIZED PEDIATRICS

The first organization that pediatricians formed in 1880 was the Section on the Diseases of Children within the AMA. The section started vigorously, but soon ran into difficulties that other budding specialties encountered within the AMA. There is no record that the section met at all in 1887 and 1888. In 1889 a resolution introduced to the AMA House of Delegates to dissolve the section was defeated, but only after an impassioned plea by the Section's chairman, J. Larrabee (Schlutz, 1933:418). In 1888, pediatricians created their own separate and independent organization, the American Pediatric Society (APS) (Pearson, 1988, 1995; Veeder, 1938, 1958). The APS technically restricted membership to researchers who had made a contribution to the understanding of childhood diseases, but with a membership of about 40, it included almost every doctor at the time with a declared interest in pediatrics (Faber and McIntosh, 1966:311; Morse, 1935:305; Pearson, 1988, 1995).

A third organization, the Association of American Teachers of the Diseases of Children (AATDC), was founded in 1907. The AATDC was instrumental in establishing pediatrics as a component of medical training. The teaching of pediatrics actually began in the 1860s when the New York Medical College allowed Abraham Jacobi to lead a weekly clinic for its students. By the end of the decade most medical schools provided some formal instruction in the treatment of children's diseases. A 1898 survey of 117 medical schools shows that only 7 (6%) offered no pediatric training. But the same survey demonstrated that few schools attached much importance to pediatrics (Griffith, 1898).

The experience of J.P. Crozer Griffith illustrates pediatrics' thwarted status in medical schools. Griffith received his medical training at the University of Pennsylvania School of Medicine during the 1870s when the school's two professors in the diseases of women also taught the diseases of children. Children got short shrift. Through Griffith's 5 years at the school only one lecture, on whooping cough, addressed the medical problems of children. In 1884 the School appointed its first professor of pediatrics, Louis Starr. But fed up with his colleagues' indifference to children, Starr resigned "in disgust" in 1891 and Griffith was appointed to replace him. He did not receive a salary for his work. He was allowed to lecture only once a week, during the last half of the final year of training. He was often assigned to the last hour of the last day of the week when students were tired and inattentive. He could not insist on attendance, nor could he set an examination (Griffith, 1936:601).

Pediatricians struggled to improve the status of pediatrics in medical schools while the medical profession was in the middle of a major overhaul in medical education. Until the beginning of the twentieth century there was little control over the quality of medical education. Some schools, particularly those affiliated with universities, stressed scientific excellence and adhered to rigorous standards. But there were many university-affiliated and commercial proprietary schools that were more concerned with profits than the adequacy of instruction or the quality of doctor they produced. In 1910, the Carnegie Foundation, in conjunction with the AMA's Council of Medical Education, commissioned Abraham Flexner to survey the state of medical education in the country.

Flexner produced a report that condemned the lack of specific entrance requirements in many medical schools and the lack of enforcement of regulations in schools that had them, the quality of teaching staff and paucity of full-time faculty, and the inadequacy of libraries (Bowers, 1976:25). Only the medical schools at Johns Hopkins University, which Flexner had used as a model against which to assess the others, Harvard University, and Western Reserve University escaped criticism. He recommended the closing of most medical schools and the

restructuring of medical education around university-based professional schools. The Flexner report revolutionized medical education in
North America. The number of schools dropped from 160 in 1905, to 95
in 1915, and 85 in 1920 (Bowers, 1976:25). The weaker schools disappeared or merged with better quality institutions. The greatest drop
was in Class C schools, the lowest category in the system the AMA's
Council on Medical Education had devised in 1906 to rate medical training programs.

The goal of the AATDC was to represent and promote the interests
of pediatricians through this process of reform. Through the organization, pediatrics made significant gains. As medical education was
redesigned, pediatrics became part of the standard medical school curriculum and as medical schools reorganized, many created independent departments of pediatrics. A survey of 42 Class A medical schools
in 1917 shows that 50% had an independent department of pediatrics
(Hess, 1917:22). By 1924, 62% of 68 Class A medical schools had an
independent department of pediatrics (Bolt, 1924:38). Besides providing
courses for medical students, pediatric departments eventually instituted postgraduate programs for those who wanted additional training.
These programs included hospital-based residencies in pediatrics and
shorter continuing education courses. In 1928, its goals realized, the
AATDC disbanded.

Throughout this period, the number of doctors with a special interest
in the problems of children grew and many of them began devoting
themselves full-time to pediatrics. That is, all of their professional activities, including teaching and research, institutional work, and private
practices, revolved exclusively around children. In 1900 there were no
more than 20 full-time pediatricians in the country. By 1914 there were
138 and by 1921 there were 664. In 1914 one out of every 1031 doctors
specialized in pediatrics. By 1921 the ratio had fallen to 1 in 218. These
figures do not include those whose practices were primarily, but not
exclusively, focused on pediatrics. There were 741 doctors in this category in 1914 and 1798 by 1921 (Table 2.2). No other specialty experienced

Table 2.2. Number of Pediatricians: 1900–1921

	1900	*1914*	*1921*
Practice limited to pediatrics	20	138	664
Special attention to pediatrics	—	741	1798
Total	—	879	2462
Ratio of pediatricians to general	—		1:1031
practitioners			1:218

Source: Veeder (1935:7).

such a rapid increase. A study of doctors who graduated between 1915 and 1920 found that while the percentage of graduates limiting themselves to surgery, internal medicine, and diseases of the eye, ear, nose, and throat had peaked and slightly declined, the percentage of those specializing in pediatrics increased nearly 100% from 5.8 in 1915 to 11.1 in 1920 (Veeder, 1935:7).

Several factors contributed to the impressive growth. One was the changing appeal of specialization, both within medicine and in the public mind. Specialties became well-paying, high status positions, popular with the middle-class public who could afford to pay for specialized care and attractive career paths for young doctors. Another factor was the increase in opportunities for pediatricians both in teaching and in practice. The expansion of pediatric departments in medical schools created new teaching positions. The proliferation of children's hospitals and special pediatric wards in general hospitals created new opportunities in the area of practice. Children's hospitals had, in the meantime, expanded from the small operations they once had been into large, complex organizations. They were no longer staffed by volunteers but by salaried, professionally trained doctors, nurses, and administrators. In 1900, there were 30 children's hospitals in the United States. By 1930, there were 70 hospitals providing 6597 patient beds (Golden, 1989; White House Conference on Child Health and Protection, 1932:23).

Finally, the child welfare movement continued to play as significant a role in pediatrics' development as it had in the specialty's emergence, and may in fact explain why pediatrics grew faster than any other specialty (Halpern, 1988). The movement had changed since its inception in the late 1800s. Before 1900 it had been concerned broadly with the conditions of childhood. After 1900 it focused on a narrower range of childhood issues, and, in particular, on infant and child mortality. Second, it had grown dramatically in size, encompassing more than 60 national organizations such as the American Association for the Study, and Prevention of Infant Mortality, the Child Health organization, and the National Child Health Council. Third, public health officials were playing a much more prominent role in the coordination and funding of child welfare activities, setting up special divisions for child health within their municipal, county and state boards of health. In 1912 the U.S. Congress established the Children's Bureau and gave it the mandate "to investigate all matters pertaining to the welfare of children and child life" (Bremner, 1971:770). But the federal Bureau's first real target was infant mortality. The strength of the movement and its success in making the issue of infant and childhood mortality a national priority boosted pediatricians' claims for recognition. In accounting for pediatrics' growth during the first decades of the twentieth century, one pediatrician (Veeder, 1935:7) wrote: "It has most certainly been due in part to the social trend of recent years, that is, to the increased sense of responsibility for the child on the part of society."

THE PEDIATRICIAN AS BABY FEEDER

While pediatricians were part of the larger movement to improve the conditions of childhood and to reduce the infant and child mortality rates, their actual contribution to that effort through the first two decades of the twentieth century was limited largely to the treatment of children's diseases. Within that already narrow mandate their concerns were more focused still on the problems associated with artificial feeding. Feeding problems dominated pediatric research, teaching, and practice from 1880 to 1920. The reasons for this emphasis lie both in the prominence of feeding problems as a source of mortality among the very young and in the context of pediatric practice during those years. Most of the serious infections that struck children were intestinal infections, and many were spread through contaminated milk. Cone (1979:152) estimates that until the 1920s, 80 to 90% of all children who died from intestinal infections were artificially fed. Most deaths occurred through the hot summer months.

These high rates of mortality are hardly surprising given the conditions under which milk was produced, handled, and distributed. Urban supplies came mostly from cows kept in dirty and cramped city stables, fed largely on garbage and distiller's mash, and often so diseased they had to be hoisted by cranes to be milked (LaFetra, 1932:38). The milk was often not only contaminated but adulterated as unscrupulous producers diluted it with water or added molasses, chalk, or plaster of Paris to improve its color (Bettman, 1974:114). George W. Goler, health inspector for the Rochester Board of Health, described the conditions of New York dairies in 1890:

> We found in many of these establishments, conditions which neither print nor pictures could adequately describe. The stables were dirty, festooned with cobwebs and badly drained; the utensils dirty, often containing layers of sour milk with admixtures of countless millions of bacteria; and the milk itself so imperfectly cared for and badly cooled that it often soured before reaching the consumer. (Bremner, 1971:871)

Working to a large extent with children who drank this milk in hospitals and other institutions, pediatricians quickly realized the disastrous consequences of artificial feeding. "To learn how to overcome this formidable cause of infant mortality," according to Cone (1979:131), "became the prime mission of pediatrics." Though an understanding of germs as a cause of disease was slowly developing through this period, pediatricians became convinced that the problem lay in the composition of cow's milk. They analyzed the precise chemical differences between cow's milk and mother's milk, and then modified cow's milk adding sugar and cream to make it a more comparable substitute. The first formulas for modification were simple. But during the 1890s Thomas Rotch developed a more complicated percentage feeding method. Rotch's method was based on the principle that no one combination of protein, fat, and carbohydrates was suited to all children. The combination depended on children's individual digestive capacities and nutritional needs. The percentages varied not only from child to child but for individual children, from week to week. The slightest variation, Rotch insisted, could make a difference in the digestibility of milk.

Rotch's method for calculating the percentages and the variations that other pediatricians introduced made the percentage feeding method increasingly complex. It took more than 20 pages in the 1903 edition of Rotch's textbook to describe it (Figure 2.1). One equation could yield up to 575 different formulas (Lawson, 1960:14). The descriptions made pediatric textbooks and journal articles look "terrifyingly like treatises on mathematics or higher astronomy" (Brenneman, 1938:65). One pediatrician (Herman F. Meyer in Cone, 1979:137) claimed the method required "almost the equivalent of an advanced degree in higher mathematics." But the percentage feeding method gave pediatricians a unique skill. "It was reserved for the skilled pediatrician," wrote L. Emmett Holt (in Evans, 1967:315), "to manage the difficult feeding case, to use the food materials of that day and with a master's touch to avoid the Scylla of indigestion and Charybdis of inanition (weakness linked to lack of nourishment)."

Not all doctors accepted the need for percentage feeding. Abraham Jacobi (1908:1219) accused advocates of the method of feeding babies "by mathematics" instead of "brains." Oliver Wendell Holmes is purported to have quipped: "A pair of substantial mammary glands has the advantage over the two hemispheres of the most learned professor's brain in the art of compounding a nutritious fluid for infants" (in Pearson, 1991:60). Moreover, subsequent research discredited the method. Faber and McIntosh (1966:52) called it "silly and dangerous," claiming it led to serious undernourishment. Others (Barness in Pearson, 1991:63) characterized the system as "absolute nonsense" and "almost gibberish." Cone (1979:137) suggests that whatever success pediatricians might have had with the formulas was probably due to their use of cleaner milk than was generally available at the time. But because the dangers of artificial feeding were so great and the correct formula was believed to make the difference between life and death, the pediatrician's esoteric expertise was highly valued. Indeed, the pediatrician's reputation as "baby-feeder" was in no small part a source of stature and legitimacy for the specialty as it was establishing itself.

> [Percentage feeding] appeared the very Eden of pediatrics, where skill was most needed and the pediatrician reigned alone and supreme. . . . Although percentage feeding has now only the importance of a historic curiosity . . . it was actually an important factor in the development of pediatrics as a specialty. Its build-up into a system of great complexity, the feeding difficulties it created, the attitude toward it akin to mysticism, and finally its grip on pediatric thought, all united to make infant feeding a subject which only the specialist of specialists could tackle. (Park and Mason, 1957:39)

The pediatrician's expert knowledge may ultimately have proven invalid. But pediatricians derived the benefit of that knowledge nevertheless as it propelled the specialty from its "ancillary status as a 'dependent dwarf' of ordinary medicine" (Cone, 1979:128), "an unwanted child in the family of medicine" (Pease, 1951:18), to one of the main branches of medicine.

DECLINING MORTALITY AND MORBIDITY

It was an unfortunate irony for pediatricians that while they established and consolidated themselves within medicine, the problems around which their specialty had first emerged were slowly disappearing. Infectious diseases began to decline around the turn of the twentieth century and continued their fall through the 1900s. For infants, the mortality rate dropped from 162.4 in 1900 to 47 in 1940 (Table 2.3 and Figure 2.2). For children aged 1 to 4 years, the rate declined from 19.8 in 1900 to 2.9 in 1940. For children aged 5 to 14, the drop was from 3.9 in 1900 to 1 in 1940 (Table 2.3 and Figure 2.3). Life expectancy, a measure of the health of the general population, increased from 47.3 in 1900 to 62.1 in 1940 (Table 2.4).

The specialty's literature leaves the impression that pediatricians had the major hand in finally conquering the threat of dreaded childhood diseases. There are references to pediatricians having "fulfilled the physician's ideal of self-elimination by doing his work so efficiently there is no longer need of him" (Powers, 1955:693). One prominent pediatrician (Levine, 1960:652) compared pediatrics to Frankenstein, "creating a

Figure 2.1. Thomas Rotch's calculations for a percentage feeding formula.

Formulae for Cream and Whey. - In order to calculate the amount of whey which is needed for various combinations, the general formulae (5), (6), and (7) can be applied by considering whey as a milk containing very low proteids (lactalbumin) and fat. Taking König's formula for whey as a standard,

Fat . . . . 0.32 = a′
Sugar . . . . 4.79 = c′
Proteids . . . . 0.86 = d′

we can then represent **a′** of the general formula by 0.32, **b′** by 0.86, and **c′** by 4.8, and the special formula will then be

(24)
$$ C = \frac{Q (0.86 \times F - 0.32 \times P)}{9.1 \text{ or } 12.6} $$

according as twelve per cent or sixteen per cent cream is used.

(25)
$$ \text{Whey} = \frac{Q F - 12 C}{0.32} \text{ or } \frac{Q F - 16 C}{0.32} $$

and

(26)
$$ L = \frac{Q 8 - (4.8 \times \text{whey} - 12 \text{ or } 16 C)}{100} $$

In such a combination sufficient diluent must be added to make up the total quantity.

The following formulae are derivable from equations expressing the fact that the proteid or fat percentage of the mixture is equal to the sum of the proteid or fat percentages contributed by the cream and the whey.

(27)
$$ P = \frac{C}{Q} \times b + \frac{\text{whey}}{Q} \times b' $$

(28)
$$ F = \frac{C}{Q} \times a + \frac{\text{whey}}{Q} \times a' $$

whence, by deduction,

(29)
$$ C = \frac{Q (F - a')}{a - a'} $$

22

One or the other of these formulae may be used according as a definite fat or proteid percentage is desired. The constants **a** and **a′** represent the fat percentages of the cream and of the whey respectively, and **b** and **b′** represent the corresponding proteid percentages.

Thus, for 20 per cent cream (F = 20, P = 3.20, S = 3.80) and whey (F = 0.32, P = 0.86, S = 4.8) the formulae would become

$$(30)\quad c = \frac{Q(P - 0.86)}{8.20 - 0.86} = (31)\ \frac{Q(P - 0.86)}{2.84}$$

and

$$(32)\quad c = \frac{Q(F - 0.32)}{20 - 0.32} = (33)\ \frac{Q(F - 0.32)}{19.68}$$

The formula for L can be derived from the general formula (7) by substitution, which gives

$$(34)\quad L = \frac{Q S - (4.8\ \text{whey} + 8.8\ C)}{100}$$

In the same way, for 16 per cent cream the formulae become, after substitution.

$$(35)\quad c = \frac{Q(P - 0.86)}{2.74}$$

$$(36)\quad c = \frac{Q(F - 0.32)}{15.08}$$

For 12 per cent cream,

$$(37)\quad c = \frac{Q(P - 0.86)}{2.94}$$

$$(38)\quad c = \frac{Q(F - 0.32)}{11.68}$$

For 8 per cent cream

$$(39)\quad c = \frac{Q(P - 0.86)}{8.01}$$

Source: Rotch (1903:236–237).

Table 2.3.   Infant, Child and Maternal Mortality Rates: 1900–1991

Year	Under 1 Year[a]	1–4 Years[b]	5–14 Years[b]	Maternal[c]
1900	162.4	19.8	3.9	—
1905	141.2	15.0	3.4	—
1910	131.8	14.0	2.9	—
1915	99.9	9.2	2.3	60.8
1920	85.8	9.9	2.6	79.9
1925	71.7	6.4	2.0	64.7
1930	64.6	5.6	1.7	67.3
1935	55.7	4.4	1.5	58.2
1940	47.0	2.9	1.0	37.6
1945	38.3	2.0	0.9	20.7
1950	29.2	1.4	0.6	8.3
1955	26.4	1.1	0.5	4.1
1960	26.0	1.1	0.5	3.7
1965	24.7	0.9	0.4	2.9
1970	20.0	0.8	0.4	2.2
1975	16.1	0.8	0.4	1.3
1980	12.6	0.7	0.4	0.9
1985	10.8	0.6	0.3	0.8
1990	9.2	0.5	0.2	0.8
1991	8.9	0.5	0.2	0.8

[a] Per 1000 live births.
[b] Per 1000 population for specified group.
[c] Per 10,000 live births.
Source: U.S. Bureau of the Census (1975:57, 60; 1985:70, 72; 1993:93; 1994:91, 95).

mechanism so efficient that it ended up by almost destroying him" Faber and McIntosh (1966:260) described pediatrics as "a suicidal specialty, bent on running itself out of business by solution of its problems."

The suggestion that pediatricians were solely or even primarily responsible for the declines is misleading. The more decisive factors were (1) better living conditions, (2) public health measures that led to improved child and maternal health, and (3) the development of preventive immunization (Dubos, 1959; McKeown, 1979; McKinlay and McKinlay, 1977). Living conditions began to improve in the second half of the nineteenth century. Public health officials did not fully or correctly comprehend the causes of infection, but they had made the connection between dirt and disease, and in what has been referred to as "the great sanitary awakening" (Winslow, 1923:12) had begun to clean up. The discovery of germs and the bacteriological revolution of the late 1800s rationalized and extended public health efforts in sanitation and led also to the epidemiological control of communicable diseases such as tuberculosis, typhoid fever, and dysentery. Using vital statistics and manda-

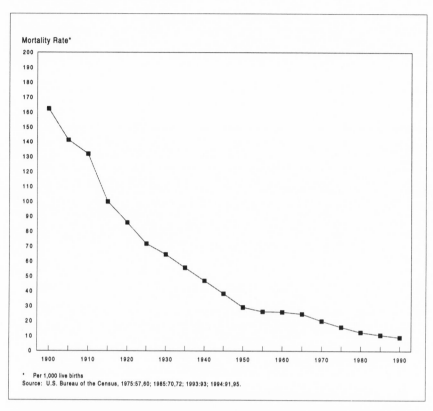

Mortality Rate*

* Per 1,000 live births
Source: U.S. Bureau of the Census, 1975:57,60; 1985:70,72; 1993:93; 1994:91,95.

Figure 2.2. Decline in infant mortality: 1900–1990. *Per 1000 live births. *Source*: U.S. Bureau of the Census (1975:57; 1985:70; 1994,91).

tory reporting ordinances, officials could trace diseases to their source and isolate or restrict the activities of carriers and their contacts.

The improvements in children's general health reduced their susceptibility to infectious diseases and better maternal health led indirectly to healthier children. The child welfare movement played the key role here as it took the latest scientific discoveries about disease prevention and translated them into effective practice. The movement's workers, mostly public health nurses and social workers, educated women through campaigns, personal visits, and special well-baby or child welfare clinics set up through the first decades of the 1900s about the value of "personal public health." They taught mothers the basic principles of child and maternal hygiene and nutrition. They promoted regular, routine medical examination for babies and instituted programs such as regular medical inspections for school children. There were also programs designed spe-

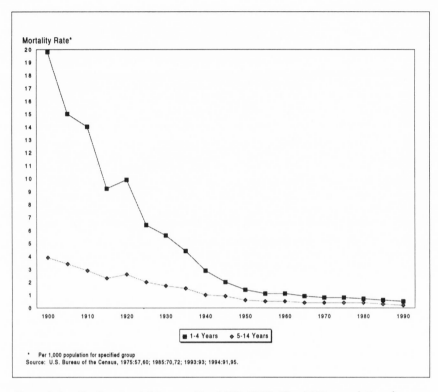

Figure 2.3. Decline in child mortality: 1900–1990. *Per 1000 population for specified group. *Source*: U.S. Bureau of the Census (1975:60; 1985:72; 1994:95).

cifically for prospective and new mothers: better screening of pregnancies to detect cases in need of specialized obstetrical care, home care
visits, and the promotion of hospital-based, as opposed to home births.
The reduction in maternal mortality after 1920 reflected improved maternal health and contributed indirectly to improved infant health. The
maternal mortality rates fell 90% from close to 80 per 100,000 live births
in 1920 to 8.3 in 1950 (Table 2.3).

Vaccines and immunizing toxoids became important in the reduction
of infant and child mortality during the 1920s. Though the idea of con-
ferring protection against life-threatening diseases had been around for
several centuries, it was not until the 1870s when Louis Pasteur developed his germ theory of disease that scientists understood how vaccines
actually worked. It took several more decades to develop safe and effective immunizing agents, in the quantities that were needed for mass
immunization, for the specific diseases that were killing children. Once

Table 2.4. Expectation of Life (in Years) at Birth: 1900–1992

1900	47.3	1925	59.0	1950	68.2	1975	72.6
1901	49.1	1926	56.7	1951	68.4	1976	72.9
1902	51.5	1927	60.7	1952	68.6	1977	73.3
1903	50.5	1928	56.8	1953	68.8	1978	73.5
1904	47.6	1929	57.1	1954	69.6	1979	73.9
1905	48.7	1930	59.7	1955	65.9	1980	73.7
1906	48.7	1931	61.1	1956	66.7	1981	74.2
1907	47.6	1932	62.1	1957	66.8	1982	74.5
1908	51.1	1933	63.3	1958	67.2	1983	74.6
1909	52.1	1934	61.1	1959	68.0	1984	74.7
1910	50.0	1935	61.7	1960	68.2	1985	74.7
1911	52.6	1936	58.5	1961	68.4	1986	74.7
1912	53.5	1937	60.0	1962	68.6	1987	74.7
1913	52.5	1938	63.5	1963	68.8	1988	74.9
1914	54.2	1939	63.7	1964	69.6	1989	75.1
1915	54.5	1940	62.9	1965	69.6	1990	75.4
1916	51.7	1941	64.8	1966	69.7	1991	75.5
1917	50.9	1942	66.2	1967	69.5	1992	75.7
1918	39.1	1943	63.3	1968	69.6		
1919	54.7	1944	65.2	1969	69.9		
1920	54.1	1945	65.9	1970	70.9		
1921	60.8	1946	66.7	1971	71.1		
1922	59.6	1947	66.8	1972	71.2		
1923	57.2	1948	67.2	1973	71.4		
1924	59.7	1949	68.0	1974	72.0		

Source: U.S. Bureau of the Census (1975:55; 1986:69; 1994:87).

the vaccines did become available public health officials set up programs to disseminate them. Vaccination became mandatory for school attendance. Educational programs for mothers of preschoolers were launched, and in many cities, municipal records were used to locate children under 5 years of age so public health nurses could reach them. The disappearance of diphtheria, pertussis, and later, polio, are directly attributable to these efforts.

LOSING THE BABY-FEEDING ROLE

For pediatrics the most consequential development was the improvement in the milk supply. By the 1890s bacteriologists knew that milk was an excellent medium for the transmission of germs and that it was the quality of milk, rather than its composition, that was most responsible for the problems surrounding the artificial feeding of infants. They had also demonstrated that pasteurization, a heat treatment that Pasteur had developed for beer and wine, could destroy harmful germs in milk. Volunteers, philanthropists, and eventually local health authorities mobilized to alert the public to the dangers of dirty milk and to make clean milk for children available. Between 1893 and 1920, hundreds of milk stations were established throughout the country. In 1907 there were 143 milk station in 24 cities across the United States; by 1915 there were 539 in 142 cities (Van Ingen, 1921:306–308). Some stations operated through the year; others operated only during the dangerous summer months.

While the milk stations dealt with the immediate problem of unsafe milk, public health officials looked for ways to safeguard the entire milk supply. Though the technology for wide-scale pasteurization was available as early as 1895, a controversy over the merits of pasteurization delayed its implementation for more than a decade. Pediatricians were among those who opposed the large-scale pasteurization of milk. They supported instead a solution that would have given pediatricians a central role in monitoring public milk supplies and possibly a new professional mission as milk-related problems declined. That solution was a system of milk certification.

Certification was developed in 1895 by Henry Leber Coit, himself a pediatrician. Visiting a local dairy to get clean milk for his dying infant son, Coit was disturbed by what he saw and began a campaign for legislative and municipal controls on milk handling. When these efforts failed he concluded that this was a task for the medical profession:

> After twenty years of experience, I believe it is hopeless to expect to bring milk up to a grade of clinical requirements by stimulating officers of the law or milk concerns, or by demands through the public press. . . . If milk fit to use for infants or for the sick is ever obtained, we must do the work necessary for its attainment ourselves. (in McCleary, 1933:62)

Coit designed a system to guarantee the quality of raw (unpasteurized) milk by assuring the quality of its source. Medical milk commissions comprised of pediatricians and other doctors certified only raw milk produced in dairies that met the commissions' strict standards. These standards covered everything from the quality of land and the construction of buildings to the care of the dairy herds and the production, transportation, and delivery of milk. The commissions also conducted regular inspections of dairies and arranged for bacteriological analyses of milk (Bremner, 1971:867–869).

Certification enjoyed a phenomenal initial success. Coit organized the first medical commission in 1892 in Essex County, New Jersey. By 1906 there were 36, and by 1912, 63 commissions across the country. In 1907 the American Association of Medical Milk Commissions and the Certified Milk Producers' Association were created to standardize regulations and methods of milk production. Pediatricians were heavily involved in the certification movement. An APS survey in 1911 showed that 26 out of 41 pediatricians sat on a medical milk commission (Carr, 1912:9). Surveys showed as well that throughout this period, most pediatricians continued to oppose pasteurization. A majority of APS members in 1898 (Waserman, 1972:372) and again in 1912 (Morse, 1935) stated that raw milk was always preferable to pasteurized milk.

To be fair, pediatricians' opposition to pasteurization was rooted in more than their professional interest in the success of certification. Though they had no way to prove it at the time, they were convinced that pasteurization altered the chemical composition of milk and destroyed some of its nutritive properties. In their private practices they had observed a rise in the incidence of scurvy among middle class children who already had access to pasteurized milk and suspected that pasteurization was to blame. Nutritionists have since established that vitamin C is indeed destroyed through pasteurization's heating process and have developed ways to fortify milk with vitamin C after pasteurization. Some pediatricians felt that wide-scale pasteurization would sanction carelessness and complacency in milk production. As they saw it, the solution to the milk problem was to produce clean milk, not to treat dirty milk.

Had the certification movement succeeded, pediatrics might have evolved into a branch of public health with special responsibility for milk production. However, after 1910 the movement faltered partly for reasons of cost—the price of a bottle of certified milk was double that of pasteurized milk—but also because it became clear that it was going to be difficult to safeguard raw milk completely. In 1909 the New York City Department of Health traced an outbreak of typhoid fever to a dairy worker who harbored the germs for typhoid fever without showing any signs of the disease (a well-carrier). In 1914 a well-carrier turned up in the herd of Coit's own model New Jersey dairy. Its efficacy in doubt, the movement began to decline, and by 1920 it had completely collapsed. As the opponents of pasteurization became less vocal and the benefits of the process more apparent, local boards of health began instituting compulsory, universal pasteurization. Chicago was the first city to require, in 1908, the pasteurization of all milk. Other communities quickly followed. The effect on intestinal infections was remarkable. According to Rosen ([1958]1993:360): "scarcely a vestige remained of the great rise in infant mortality that generally came with the hot weather."

The availability of clean milk was not the only factor responsible for the pediatrician's disappearing baby-feeding role. By the 1920s safe and easy to use commercially manufactured infant food formulas became available and were skillfully marketed by their producers. Mothers who could not breast feed their babies, as well as those who no longer wished to, started to use the formulas (Apple, 1980). Even pediatricians frustrated with the complexity of the percentage method found the products attractive. One of them (Darley, 1911:747) admitted: "It is no wonder that many busy practitioners have given up the whole [feeding] problem in despair and have resorted to the use of the patent baby foods as the easiest way out of the difficulty."

Pediatricians did not relinquish their baby feeding function passively. As in the case of certification, they attempted to salvage a role for themselves in artificial feeding. As the popularity of the formulas grew, pediatricians struck a deal with manufacturers that allowed them to control the information needed to use the new products (Apple, 1980, 1987). The manufacturers, recognizing that they could neutralize medical opposition to their products by giving the medical profession an interest in their use, stopped advertising directly to the public and geared their campaigns toward doctors instead. As Apple (1980:417) puts it: "Manufacturers sold, but medical practitioners controlled: a mutually advantageous relationship between physicians and infant food companies had been established." Thus, pediatricians continued to advise and supervise the artificial feeding of young children. But baby feeding was certainly not the complicated task it once had been. Brenneman (1933:9–10), a pediatrician who had once used the percentage method, captured the lost aura:

> The pediatrician is today actually embarrassed at times in deciding which one of so many simple ways of feeding a baby to choose in a given case. . . . A surgeon once asked me: "What are you feeding babies *today*? and I could not logically resent the implication.

Once the source of such status and pride for the pediatrician, baby feeding had become an embarrassment and source of derision.

THE SHIFT INTO PREVENTION

As they witnessed not only the loss of the pediatrician's baby feeding role but the general declines in mortality and morbidity, the specialty's leaders began to take a dim view of its future. Borden Veeder, president of the APS in 1935, delivered an address to the organization that sounded like a eulogy for a dying specialty. Veeder felt that with the disappearance of so many infectious childhood diseases and the incorporation of pediatrics into medical school training, general practitioners could take over most child health care. Pediatrics, as a specialized area of practice, he predicted, was headed for an irreversible decline: "The pediatrician, as he exists in practice today and as he has developed so rapidly in the last few years," he wrote, "will find the need and opportunity for him rapidly diminishing. . . . The trend towards specialization in pediatrics will decrease." "Above all," he continued, "young medical men must not be encouraged to enter blindly into a field of practice which, as it at present exists, is rapidly becoming limited in its opportunities and future" (Veeder, 1935:9–10).

Another leading pediatrician, John L. Morse, in his address to the Philadelphia Pediatric Society on its fortieth anniversary in 1937 was also pessimistic. "I am quite certain," he said (Morse, 1937:532), "that the lot of pediatricians has been much better in the last forty years than it will be in the next forty. . . . It is evident that the opportunities for pediatricians will not be as great in the future as they have been in the past. Forty years ago, pediatrics was a virgin field; now it is overcultivated." He facetiously suggested that young doctors pursue careers in geriatrics rather than pediatrics:

The other end of life now offers the greatest field of development. There are more old people than there used to be, and almost all of them are ill in some way, or, at any rate, are wearing out; they like many visits; they are more interesting than children; the doctor is not blamed when they die; and the estate pays the bill. . . . My advice to young physicians is, therefore, to take up geriatrics, not pediatrics. (Morse, 1937:532)

The predictions were wrong, or at least premature. Pediatrics did not decline, it flourished. The number of pediatricians increased from 689 in 1923 to 6567 in 1955. The specialty's rate of growth far outstripped that of both other specialties and doctors in general (Table 2.5). Such growth

Table 2.5. Medical Manpower Trends: 1923–1962

Year	Pediatricians	Specialists	Total Number of Doctors
1923	689	15,408	145,966
1938	2,205	33,618	169,629
1949	4,315	62,688	201,277
1955	6,567	84,441	218,061
1962	10,507	129,838	257,035
Percent increase 1923–1962	1,425	743	76

Source: Adapted from Stewart and Pennell (1963:316).

was possible because during the 1920s pediatricians began to offset the diminishing need for their expertise in artificial feeding and the treatment of disease with preventive care.

Though the importance of disease prevention had been part of pediatricians' rhetoric since the inception of the specialty, preventive care up until the 1920s had never been a major part of routine pediatric practice. Pediatrics' foray into routine health maintenance started with their work in the well-child clinics set up to instruct mothers in basic child hygiene. While the original purpose of the clinics had been educational, through the 1920s they hired pediatricians to provide routine examinations as part of the "well-child conference" or visit. The clinics also stressed the need to have the growth and development of healthy children monitored regularly by a pediatrician.

The high profile that the clinic workers gave pediatricians and the educational campaigns launched by the child welfare movement created a growing demand for preventive child care services. The movement had established the clinics primarily for the lower and immigrant classes who had a higher rate of infant mortality than the rest of the population. But with the success of their campaigns, mothers of all classes were flocking to the clinics clamoring for routine check-ups for their children. Middle class mothers increasingly sought, and were willing to pay for, the same services from private doctors. They found that general practitioners, by and large, did not really see preventive work as part of their role as doctors, and were, therefore, not eager to do check-ups. Pediatricians, on the other hand, were obliging. Many of them were used to doing such check-ups in the clinics. It was a small step to provide the same services in their private practices. Moreover, they discovered that if they were willing to combine their treatment of sick children with the supervision of healthy children, they could make full-time careers out of private practice without having to add teaching or institutional work. As more of them were drawn to this option, pediatrics began to evolve into a largely primary care specialty (Halpern, 1988).

The shift into prevention and primary care brought with it a new pediatric organization. Those who were in full-time, primary care practices eventually felt that there was no group within the specialty to speak on their behalf. The APS, since its creation in 1888, had become an increasingly more exclusive scientific society limiting its membership to those with an established record of pediatric teaching and research. In fact, even younger academically inclined pediatricians, frustrated by their lack of access to the APS, formed the Society for Pediatric Research (SPR) in 1932 and restricted membership to researchers under 45 years of age. As the number of primary care pediatricians grew, they initially gravitated toward the AMA's Section on the Diseases of Children as an organizational locus. There was also talk of expanding the APS to accommodate them. But primary care pediatricians finally decided to create their own organization and in 1929 the American Academy of Pediatrics (AAP) was formed.

Through the AAP primary care pediatricians mobilized to promote their interests in prevention (Halpern, 1988). This involved two strategies: First, they sought to eliminate the threat posed by the public, well-child clinics. After they began offering preventive services in their private practices, primary care pediatricians began to criticize the clinic system. They argued that the clinics were inadequate because within the context of the clinics they saw children in isolation without prior knowledge of their full medical histories, nor of their normal, everyday surroundings. Constant turnover in personnel was another problem since it meant that children were not getting continuity of care. They insisted as well, that the clinics would never be able to satisfy the health care needs of the entire child population (Veeder, 1922:2228–2229).

Through the 1920s primary care pediatricians tolerated the clinics, at least for those who could not afford private doctors. They made an issue only out of the clientele that the clinics attracted and their use by the well-to-do. They succeeded in the late 1920s in getting some clinics to place restrictions on services on the basis of family income. But by the time the AAP was formed in 1929 they were determined to close the clinics altogether. When the bill providing congressional funding for the clinics came up for renewal in 1930 in the form of the Jones–Bankhead Act, pediatricians withheld their support. Though their equivocation was not the only factor in the bill's ultimate defeat, it did contribute to it. Without funding, the well-child clinics could not survive. At their height in 1930 there had been over 4000 such clinics scattered throughout the country (White House Conference on Child Health and Protection, 1932). By 1945 the clinic system had collapsed giving pediatricians a virtual monopoly on preventive child health care.

The second strategy in securing the interests of primary care pediatricians was the development of a system to certify doctors with pediatric training. As a result of the campaigns of the child welfare movement, the public already connected prevention with pediatricians. But there were no controls over standards of training, nor, more importantly, over who could use the title "pediatrician." Pediatricians feared that as the demand for preventive services increased, more doctors, including general practitioners with no background in pediatrics beyond their undergraduate training, would lay claim to the title. Other specialties, facing similar problems, were developing a mechanism to identify those with specialty training. They created boards that set standards of specialty training, conducted examinations, and issued certificates to those who qualified. The specialty boards did not keep anyone from limiting their practice to a particular area. But they did restrict the use of the specialist label. The American Board of Ophthalmology was the first such board that was formed in 1916, followed by the American Boards of Obstetrics-Gynecology in 1930 and Dermatology in 1932 (Geyman, 1971:4). A spate of others were created through the 1930s.

Once the AAP was created, it began to organize such a board for pediatrics. Under its initiative, representatives of all the three major pediatric organizations (AAP, APS, AMA Section on the Diseases of Children) met in 1933 and established the American Board of Pediatrics (ABP). The ABP ruled that all applicants for certification had to complete a 3 year residency in pediatrics. Between 1933 and 1938, the ABP issued over 1200 certificates to qualifying pediatricians (Faber and McIntosh, 1966:193).

PEDIATRIC SUBSPECIALTIES

There was a final development that set the stage for the "dissatisfied pediatrician syndrome" of the 1950s—and that was the creation of pediatric subspecialties. The subspecialties grew out of a series of specialized clinics and outpatient units that the pediatric departments of medical schools and teaching hospitals had started to set up through the 1930s. Rather than providing general medical services to sick children, the clinics focused on particular problem areas such as allergies, hormonal disorders, heart conditions, and epilepsy. These problems, then as now, were relatively rare among children and pediatric educators felt that by bringing as many cases as possible in one place they would facilitate research and the development of effective treatment.

The clinics were staffed by pediatricians with special research interests in these areas. The first subspecialists typically combined their work in the clinics with private, general pediatric practices and/or with academic duties. By the 1940s many were building full-time careers in subspecialties. They acquired advanced training in these areas early in their careers either to secure full-time academic and hospital positions that allowed them to teach and research or to set themselves up as hospital-based consulting subspecialists working by referral. While the majority of pediatricians were building primary care practices in preventive work and general pediatrics then, these pediatricians were committing themselves to more specialized areas of care.

Inevitably the subspecialists began to identify less with general pediatrics and more with those colleagues who shared their more focused interests. In much the same way that the first pediatricians came together to create their specialty, these subspecialists formed their own professional institutions, published their own journals, set up their own sections within general pediatric organizations such as the APS, the SPR, and the AAP, and eventually created their own independent organizations. By the 1950s there were even subspecialty certifying boards designating subspecialists as the preferred providers of pediatric services within their fields. In 1951, a Subboard of Pediatric Allergy was formed. In 1960, the Subboard of Pediatric Cardiology came into existence. Over the 1960s and 1970s subboards in pediatrics endocrinology, pediatric gastroenterology, pediatric hematology–oncology, pediatric infectious diseases, pediatric nephology, neonatal–perinatal medicine, pediatric pulmonology, pediatric rheumatology, pediatric critical care medicine, and pediatric emergency medicine (jointly with the American Board of Emergency Medicine) were also established (*Official ABMS Directory of Board Certified Medical Specialists*, 1994:4667). By the 1950s, general or primary care pediatricians were recognizing the limitations of their own skills in treating serious childhood illnesses and referring difficult cases to these subspecialists.

Chapter 3

The Dissatisfied Pediatrician Syndrome

INTRODUCTION

The 1950s should have been a high point in pediatric history. The difficult battles for recognition had been fought and won. The specialty had established and consolidated itself organizationally. The potential crisis created by the disappearance of baby-feeding as a problem and the improved health of children had been averted with the move into prevention. Moreover, birth rates had jumped dramatically in the post-World War II period, creating a huge demand for pediatric services. Between 1946 and 1956, the birth rate climbed almost 20% from 20.4 to 24.1 per 1000 population. It rose another 10% to 26.6 per 1000 in 1957 and continued to hover around 25 until the end of the decade (Table 3.1). Primary care pediatricians had so successfully built a reputation as child health experts that most of this demand was directed their way rather than toward general practitioners. In fact, there were predictions that pediatricians would one day monopolize child health care entirely: general practice would eventually disappear and primary care pediatricians would, in effect, become general practitioners among the young.

Instead the specialty faced a crisis so severe some pediatricians were asking themselves whether primary care pediatrics would survive. Within pediatric circles the crisis was referred to as the "dissatisfied pediatrician syndrome" (Vandersall, 1963). The term described a profound and pervasive sense of malaise and disaffection among primary care pediatricians. Their complaints covered a range of issues. But the major problem was the lack of challenge and stimulation in pediatric practice. The dissatisfied pediatrician syndrome was pivotal in the emergence of the new pediatrics because it was in the context of the debate it generated that some pediatricians first began to suggest that perhaps if the specialty were to extend its mandate beyond physical complaints, practitioners might find the challenges they were seeking.

What brought on the dissatisfied pediatrician syndrome and why did the specialty experience such a crisis during what should have been yet

38   The Dissatisfied Pediatrician Syndrome

Table 3.1.   Live Birth and Birth Rates: 1945–1991

Year	Live Births[a]	Birth Rate[b]	Year	Live Births	Birth Rate
1945	2,858	20.4	1969	3,600	17.8
1946	3,411	24.1	1970	3,731	18.4
1947	3,817	26.6	1971	3,556	17.2
1948	3,637	24.9	1972	3,258	15.6
1949	3,649	24.5	1973	3,137	14.8
1950	3,632	24.1	1974	3,160	14.8
1951	3,823	24.9	1975	3,144	14.6
1952	3,913	25.1	1976	3,168	14.6
1953	4,965	25.0	1977	3,327	15.1
1954	4,078	25.3	1978	3,333	15.0
1955	4,104	25.0	1979	3,494	15.6
1956	4,218	25.2	1980	3,612	15.9
1957	4,308	25.3	1981	3,629	15.8
1958	4,255	24.5	1982	3,681	15.9
1959	4,245	24.0	1983	3,639	15.6
1960	4,258	23.7	1984	3,669	15.6
1961	4,268	23.3	1985	3,761	15.8
1962	4,167	22.4	1986	3,757	15.6
1963	4,098	21.7	1987	3,809	15.7
1964	4,027	21.0	1988	3,910	16.0
1965	3,760	19.4	1989	4,041	16.4
1966	3,606	18.4	1990	4,158	16.7
1967	3,521	17.8	1991	4,111	16.3
1968	3,502	17.5			

[a] In thousands.
[b] Live births per 1,000 population.
Source: U.S. Bureau of the Census (1975:49; 1985:56; 1994:76).

another period of continued growth and prosperity? These are the questions that this chapter explores. At the heart of the dissatisfied pediatrician syndrome were changes in the nature of private, primary care pediatric practices after 1950. Prevention at first only supplemented the pediatrician's role in treating disease. By 1950, however, prevention was dominating pediatric practice. At the same time the nature of childhood morbidity was changing dramatically. Through the 1930s and 1940s, even though many of the major childhood killers of the previous century had been eliminated, there were still serious childhood infections and diseases for the pediatrician to treat. By 1950 the threat of even many of these diseases was disappearing, and what serious illness remained required the services of the pediatric subspecialists who were coming on to the scene. The result was that primary care pediatricians were spending most of their time either supervising the growth and development of children who were healthy or seeing children with minor, easily treated, and often entirely self-correcting medical problems. The reasons for these trends and their impact on pediatric primary care practice are discussed below.

THE GROWTH IN PREVENTION AND ROUTINE CARE

The growth in preventive and routine care as a component of pediatric primary care practices was the outcome primarily of the development of disease-fighting drugs. In 1935 Gerhard Domagk, a German organic chemist, synthesized sulfanilamide, a compound that could fight a range of infections in the human body by impairing the ability of harmful germs to reproduce. Over the next 5 years, hundreds of other sulfa drugs were synthesized, giving doctors the first real weapon they had against infections. But as scientists soon realized, the sulfa drugs were not a panacea. Some seemed to interfere with the body's natural defense against infection, while others stimulated the production of sulfa-resistant strains of germs.

Through the 1940s the sulfa drugs were superseded by penicillin. Penicillin was first discovered by Alexander Fleming in 1928. But Fleming had difficulty purifying his new discovery. The excitement over the sulfa drugs through the 1930s delayed further progress until 1940, when Howard F. Florey and Ernest B. Chain succeeded in isolating it and developing it for clinical use. Through the 1940s and early 1950s a host of other antibiotics with germ-fighting potential stronger and wider than penicillin were developed, including streptomycin, chlortetracycline, chloramphenicol, the cephalosporins, oxytetracycline, and tetracycline. Drug companies launched large scale production immediately. By 1950, they were manufacturing over 400 tons of antibiotics annually (Welch, 1958:77).

Both the sulfonamides and antibiotics were a boon to medical practice and, especially, to pediatrics, because infections among children, though not as rampant as they had been before public health measures had been introduced, were still prevalent. The availability of effective medical treatment meant that the drop in mortality rates that had started earlier in the century continued just as precipitously through the 1940s and 1950s. For infants the rates between 1935 and 1960 dropped from 55.7 to 26.4 per 1000 live births; for children in the 1–4 year age category the decline was from 4.4 to 1.1 per 1000 (see Table 2.3); and for children between 5 and 14 years of age, the figures are 1.5 and 0.5 per 1000 (see Table 2.3). Much of this decline is attributable to the reduction in the number of deaths due to scarlet fever and pneumonia, which public health measures had not been successful in controlling.

Besides eliminating the threat of scarlet fever and pneumonia, the sulfonamides and antibiotics simplified and routinized the treatment of many other infections, which, while not necessarily life-threatening, were still dangerous. Indeed, they almost eliminated the need for a firm diagnosis. It became common practice for pediatricians to prescribe antibiotics for several days without examining the child carefully, and then trying to diagnose only those for whom the treatment did not work. "Many a physician," observed one pediatrician (Washburn, 1951:304), "conscientious enough but with a heavy practice load—has found it far too easy to give maximum doses of penicillin, streptomycin, etc., without even bothering to establish a diagnosis other than that the child was obviously ill with a high temperature." The practice was condemned by pediatric instructors, but even they admitted that it was usually effective and rarely caused harm (Davison, 1952:537).

THE CHANGING COMPOSITION OF PEDIATRIC PRACTICE

A series of studies in the pediatric literature make it possible to trace the growth of prevention and routine care as a component of pediatric practice after 1930 (Table 3.2). The studies are not entirely comparable. Some provide a snapshot view of a pediatric practice at a particular point in time, and others look longitudinally at changes in practice patterns over time; some focus on private or small, group practices while others survey the specialty at large at a city, regional, or national level. Moreover, the categories used to classify the range of problems treated and

Table 3.2. Distribution of Patient Visits Between Well-Care and Disease

Author	Years Surveyed	Well-care (%)	Disease (%)
Aldrich (1934)	1933–1934	39	61
London (1937)	1937	39	61
Geppert (1958)	1946–1952	32	68
Boulware (1958)	1930–1955	40	60
AAP (1950)	1950	54	46
Deisher et al. (1960)	1958	49	51
Jacobziner et al. (1962)	1958–1959	57	41
Breese et al. (1966)	1959–1960	39	61
Bergman et al. (1966)	1964	50	50
Hessel/Haggerty (1968)	1966	49	51
Mean	Before 1952	40	60
Mean	After 1952	49	51

Source: Adapted from Hessel and Haggerty (1968:276).

services provided are not the same across studies. Despite these limitations, the studies provide a general picture of the changing trends. They
show the extent to which preventive work sustained primary care pediatric practices after 1930 and how prevention grew as a component of
pediatric practice.

One of the first composition studies appeared in 1934 and describes
the private practice of C. Anderson Aldrich in Winnetka, Illinois. Aldrich (1934) is not clear about the time period his records cover, indicating only that they extend back over "the past few years." The records
show clearly, however, that 39% of all the cases that Aldrich treated
involved what he referred to as the routine care of infants (prescribing
formulas, handling teething difficulties, cultivating appetite, and wean-
ing), routine examination of children 1 year of age and over, and preventive treatment (vaccination and immunization). The remaining 61%
involved treatment for such conditions as upper respiratory infections
(23%), other acute infectious diseases (22%), and gastrointestinal disorders (4%).

Arthur H. London (1937), a practitioner in Durham, North Carolina,
recorded that of the first 1500 children he had ever treated since starting
his practice, 39% required only routine or preventive care. J.R. Boulware
(1958) compared the records of his Lakeland, Florida practice over the
period 1930–1955 to Aldrich's study using Aldrich's original system of
categorization. His tables show that 40% of all the cases he had managed
over the 25-year period entailed routine and preventive care. Though
none of these studies captures longitudinal trends, Boulware (1958:555)
did comment tellingly on the changing character of pediatric practice
over the course of his career: "Practice in the early years consisted of
difficult feeding problems, preventive injections and the time-consum-
ing treatment of children severely ill with such diseases as lobar pneumonia, empyema, infectious colitis and diphtheria. Now there is a
greater percentage of time devoted to well-baby care, and general health
conferences."

By 1950 the percentage of preventive work alone had grown even
higher to at least 50% of all cases. Several surveys, as well as analyses of
individual practices, reflected the trend. An AAP (1950) national survey
showed that 54% of all visits to pediatricians were for health supervision;
only 46% were for the care of sick children. A state-wide survey of
Washington pediatricians in 1958 (Deisher, Derby, and Sturman, 1960)
showed that they spent 49% of their time doing well-child care as opposed to 51% doing sick-child care. The same survey revealed, ironically
though not surprisingly, that general practitioners were more likely to
treat sick children in the pediatric components of their practices than were
pediatricians. Seventy-one percent of all pediatric care that general practi-

tioners provided consisted of treatment for illness, while only 29% involved well-child care. In New York City 57% of all visits to pediatricians by children under 6 years of age involved well-child care; 43 involved the treatment of sick children (Jacobziner, Rich, and Mercant, 1962). The corresponding figures for general practitioners are 31% for well-child care and 69% for disease treatment. Among 19 pediatricians in Monroe County, New York, 49% of patient visits had to do with well-child care while 51% involved sick-child care (Hessel and Haggerty, 1968).

Figures for individual practices were for the most part consistent. In a time-motion study of four pediatricians in Seattle, Washington, in which their activities over five nonsuccessive days in 1964 were carefully followed and recorded, Bergman, Dassel, and Wedgwood (1966) found that they spent 50% of their time in well-child care. The next largest category of activity involved respiratory infections, which consumed 22% of the time. The authors of the study noted that none of the pediatricians encountered a single case of serious disease over the 5 days they were observed. The sickest patient was a child with a persistent case of croup. The pediatrician decided to hospitalize the child, but only as a precaution. A study of a three-pediatrician practice in Brighton, a residential community outside of Rochester, New York, produced the only aberrant results, though the amount of preventive work was still high at 39% (Breese, Disney, and Talpey, 1966).

When the proportions of well-child to sick-child care in the pre- and post-1950 studies are averaged, there is an increase of almost 10% from 40 to 49% in the distribution of visits for well-child care and a corresponding decrease from 60 to 51% in the distribution of visits for sick child care. The figures capture numerically the observation that medical historian William Smillie made when he compared the health prospects of children in 1950 to those of children in 1850:

> The picture has entirely changed in 100 years. . . . Every single one of the ten important causes of illness and death in infancy and early childhood in 1850 has been wiped out. The slate is clean. Childhood has become a period of abundant health and of preparation for a full and satisfactory adult life, free from invalidism and from the scars of early acute infections. (Smillie, 1955:207)

For primary care pediatricians then, the changing child health picture meant that there were far fewer sick children to treat. Most simply required well-child care. Those who were ill suffered from relatively minor conditions that either resolved themselves without any treatment or could be easily treated by a doctor who did not really need the specialized skills of a pediatrician. But when, or more accurately, if, a seriously ill child did appear, the primary care pediatrician was usually not the best equipped to handle the case, and the child would be referred to the better qualified subspecialist. The dissatisfied pediatrician syndrome indicated that a growing number of pediatricians were not content with this pattern of practice.

EXPRESSIONS OF DISCONTENT

The dissatisfied pediatrician syndrome started with "vague rumblings of discontent" (May, 1959:253) among primary care pediatricians and assertions that the specialty simply did not offer the rewards it once had. By the end of the 1950s it had escalated into an open discussion of a range of problems. Pediatric journals were deluged with letters of complaint. The letters spoke of long hours, overwhelming work loads, fatigue, and poor remuneration. The income of pediatricians was, in fact, comparatively low. Since preventive and routine services typically generate less income than treatment, and since so much of pediatric practice consisted of such services, pediatricians earned less than any other major specialty and barely more than general practitioners. A 1959 survey (*Medical Economics*, 1961:90) showed that the net earnings of pediatricians averaged 20,700 dollars, compared to 22,300 for specialists in internal medicine, 24,300 for psychiatrists, 24,800 for dermatologists, 24,800 for ophthalmologists, 25,900 for otolaryngologists, 27,900 for obstetricians/gynecologists, 27,900 for general surgeons, and 32,700 for orthopedic surgeons. The net earnings of pediatricians was only about 700 dollars more than that of general practitioners at 20,000 (Table 3.3).

Table 3.3. Net Earnings for General Practice and Nine Specialties: 1959

Specialty	Net Income
Orthopedic surgery	32,700
General surgery	27,900
Obstetrics/gynecolocy	27,900
Otolaryngology	25,900
Dermatology	24,800
Ophthalmology	24,800
Internal medicine	22,300
Psychiatry	20,700
Pediatrics	20,700
General practice	20,000
All specialties	24,800

Source: Medical Economics (1961:90).

Table 3.4.   Net Earnings[a] for All Doctors and Selected Specialties: 1965–1970

Speciality	1965	1966	1967	1968	1969	1970
All medical doctors	28.9	32.1	34.7	37.6	40.5	41.5
General surgery	32.5	35.6	37.7	40.7	42.9	45.0
Obstetrics/gynecology	30.5	33.9	37.4	39.7	43.8	47.0
Internal medicine	27.7	32.3	32.5	38.8	38.4	41.3
General practice	25.1	27.7	31.4	32.9	35.1	37.4
Pediatrics	25.2	28.1	27.6	32.9	34.4	35.9

[a] In thousands of dollars.
Source: U.S. Bureau of the Census (1972:68).

The disparities in income levels between pediatricians and other doctors became even more pronounced through the 1960s. In 1967, general practitioners actually outranked pediatricians in net earnings: pediatricians earned on average only 27,600 dollars compared to general practitioners, who earned 31,400. In 1968, the net earnings of the two groups were comparable at 32,900 dollars. But in 1969, and again in 1970, general practitioners overtook pediatricians (Table 3.4).

Yet figures for the same period showed that pediatricians worked longer hours and saw more patients than the average doctor. In 1965, 39% of pediatricians reported working 70 hours or more per week, in comparison to 17.5% for all doctors. Only 8% of pediatricians reported working 49 hours per week or less, in comparison to 26% for all doctors (Table 3.5). Pediatricians averaged 3 home visits, 116 office visits, and 17 hospital visits per week, while other doctors averaged 1 home visit, 87 office visits, and 17 hospital visits (Table 3.6).

But what these letters captured most vividly was the agonizing frustration that pediatricians were experiencing in their practices. They longed for the challenge and intellectual excitement of treating serious childhood illnesses. Instead, their long days were filled with routine check-ups and minor, easily treated, if not self-correcting illnesses.

Table 3.5.   Working Hours per Week for Pediatricians and All MDs: 1965

	Pediatricians	All Doctors
70 or more	39.1	17.5
60–69	36.8	28.0
50–59	16.1	28.4
49 or less	8.0	26.1

Source: White (1965).

Table 3.6. Patient Visits per Week to Pediatricians and All MDs: 1965

Type	Pediatricians	All Doctors
Home visits	3	1
Office visits	116	87
Hospital visits	17	17

Source: White (1965).

Some had left pediatrics for other areas of medical practice; others were considering leaving. The letters were a powerful expression of the disaffection among the ranks of general primary care pediatricians. They are worth quoting at length.

One of the first letters published was written by Frank L. Tabrah (1957). Tabrah had graduated from the University of Buffalo Medical School in 1943. After completing a pediatric residency at the Buffalo Children's Hospital and Children's Orthopedic Hospital in Seattle, he set up a private pediatric practice in Bellingham, Washington where he remained until 1956. In that year, fed up with what he referred to as the tedium of "playing grandmother" for years on end, Tabrah gave up his practice and joined the staff of the medical department in the Kohala Sugar Company, in Kohala, Hawaii. He wrote a long, thoughtful, and provocative letter explaining his reasons for leaving pediatrics.

Pediatrics, during the first half of this century, has been a brilliant part of our whirlwind social advance. Improved infant feeding, the abolition of the contagious scourges, and the understanding of growth and development have, with the coming of fantastic surgical techniques, been sufficient to nearly eliminate the need for large numbers of pediatricians.

Rapid transportation and antibiotics have revolutionized our work. Gone is the day when it took a genius to feed a normal infant—our earlier gems of knowledge and techniques have fortunately become almost public knowledge. The rising level of education has made the ordinary routine of providing for an infant fairly simple. . . .

Rapid social and economic changes, particularly the way in which medicine is actually practiced, will often surprise and dismay the recent newcomer to pediatrics. Since the specialties have arrived, even in small towns, and especially the subspecialties in pediatrics, cardiology, radiology, otolaryngology, surgery (orthopedic, etc.), the pediatrician is indeed low man on the totem pole, his position comparable to that in which the general practitioner imagines himself, but without the satisfactions and interests of the generalist's broad attack on the whole of medical practice, not to mention his income from surgery and obstetrics. Well babies still frequent the pediatrician's office, but it is inconceivable that any physician with intelligence and interest in the usual can long survive the routine of playing grandmother for years on end in a well-baby practice.

A few years ago this colorless job was relieved by challenges of frequent and severe disease, and the physician was continually called upon to exercise his greatest ingenuity. He felt deep satisfaction in his work, a satisfaction which is waning today because of the changed nature of our practice, except in large centers where unusual cases congregate.

My former pediatric practice in a Northwest city is a good example. With a population of about 60,000, well supplied with competent general practitioners and top quality specialists, the daily routine was monotonous in the extreme. Upper respiratory infections, infant feeding, the endless discussions with endless mothers of problems that are self-righting anyhow—all of it except the occasional emergency situation was not sufficiently stimulating for a steady diet. There are no longer enough surprises in the package. . . . If the specialty is to continue unchanged, extreme care will be needed to make certain that those intending to do only pediatric office practice are aware of its enforced preoccupation with trivia largely unrelated to disease.

Few men will knowingly accept such a career—in time the specialty may lose the top quality men it has attracted in past years. The intern who contemplates a career in pediatric medicine must, I believe, be willing to look for realistic satisfaction in his work in one of two ways, either in the teaching hospital where he can well use the bulk of his training, or in some consultative position requiring knowledge of the field of pediatric medicine, such as public health planning or in some work such as assisting with hospital development in foreign countries, or full-time research. Pediatric medical office practice is not enough; there are too many private pediatric practices being started today that will be abandoned from sheer boredom. (Tabrah, 1957:745–746)

Tabrah's letter was a catalyst, sparking an avalanche of similar admissions. Thornton Vandersall (1963), a pediatrician in Long Island, New York, wrote about the disenchantment he felt with his specialty choice once in practice, and his efforts to try to recapture the enthusiasm for pediatrics he had experienced as a resident. When these efforts failed, he too, after only 3 years in practice, made the decision to leave pediatrics and retrain in psychiatry.

One year age, after three years in practice, I left pediatrics and began a 3-year fellowship in psychiatry. In the belief that my thoughts about leaving have more than purely personal validity, I am submitting them here.

I began with the stark realization that I did not like practice. Having reveled in hospital pediatrics, I was surprised. I first complained that the work of practice [well-baby care] was not essential compared to "sick child" care in hospital. Any mother who picks up the phone to call a pediatrician can point out the error in that argument. I further reasoned: perhaps it is essential, but to me it is dull and routine. . . .

I thought first of the original choice on leaving medical school. I chose to take care of, and was well trained to take care of, sick children. Three busy and important years were invested in this. Of course I had work in well baby care, but my interest was never fully there and no one forced me to the point where I was stimulated to a true interest in well children and parents. On entering practice I found that I was not trained for what I was doing. With the help of colleagues in a group I spent about six months mastering the new task. Then I experienced ennui and some other feeling all too familiar to the practitioner.

My next step consisted of additional familiar maneuvers. These might be called "attempts to reclaim the lost glory." They consisted of such things as returning to the "center" one day a week to be the 99th wheel, reading the journals so that I could discuss the pathology that I rarely saw, and spicing my conversation with that one annual "good case of _____." Although this behavior now seems almost irrational to me, it was the familiar ex-resident pattern.

Sooner or later we must realize that we have made a major intellectual, physical, and emotional investment in the treatment and understanding of serious organic pathology and that we simply are not working in that area. Because we are not trained for, and do not understand tasks that are presented to us, we end frustrated, discontented and angry. Our self-presentation as the healer is irreparably compromised. There are truly few to heal, but many to tend. (Vandersall, 1963:465)

Kenneth Gould (1964) was a graduate of New York University College of Medicine and trained in pediatrics at Bellevue and Kings County Hospitals, and in hematology at Children's Hospital of Michigan. After almost 8 years in private pediatric practice, he, like Vandersall, decided to leave and become a psychiatrist. His contact with colleagues who were going through the same turmoil convinced him that his experience was not isolated. They had all shared an initial commitment to, and passion for, their specialty, which dissipated once they were in private practice.

My reasons for this decision [to leave] were many and varied. I felt that most of them were unique with me. However, as I have continued my training in psychiatry I have met several other pediatricians who have taken a similar course, and surprisingly enough, characteristics common to us have emerged. We all found the experience of hospital pediatrics exciting, challenging, and rewarding in a personal and professional way. We enjoyed the wards, the children, the families of our patients, and probably above all, the feeling of accomplishment. The private practice of pediatrics was looked forward to with pleasure and anticipation. Peculiarly enough it seems that most of us did not question whether private practice was similar to residency work. We loved children. They were enjoyable to work with, and there was a lot to accomplish with them. The features of private practice in pediatrics in most cases were neither shown nor discussed with us. We were sitting on top of a very happy professional cloud. (Gould, 1964:790)

Gould went on to describe how his first few years in practice were busy getting established and building a patient base. Eventually he took on two associates. But all of them found, despite their success, that they were not satisfied with their professional lives:

The problems are fairly well known to most practitioners. The heavy case load, the majority of visits concerning well-baby care and simple self-limited respiratory and gastrointestinal illnesses, the oppressive telephone, the frequent nights and weekends on, and the relatively low remuneration for such work present real difficulties. (Gould, 1964:790)

Gould ended his letter by expressing his reservations about the future of pediatrics as a specialty:

I have written this letter because I am deeply concerned with the future of American pediatrics. I do not believe that pediatrics can survive in the direction it is going. There must be an "agonizing reappraisal" of the future of private pediatric practice in this country. . . .

These difficulties that present a crisis to our specialty (I can't bring myself to say "former specialty") must be discussed, rediscussed and finally solved within the profession. . . . If this is not done, the future of private pediatric practice in America is indeed gloomy. (Gould, 1964:790–791)

R. Dean Coddington, a pediatrician from Red Bank, New Jersey, experienced his dilemma as a double-bind. On the one hand, he pointed out, there was the temptation to relieve the oppressive boredom of routine care by encouraging mothers to become more independent and confident about their mothering skills so that they would be able to deal with most of their children's problems on their own. But without the broad range of problems that mothers typically brought to the pediatrician, few pediatricians, especially those just starting their practices and eager for a stable client base, would be able to survive in private practice.

First of all, a conflict of interests arises in the young pediatrician's mind when on the one hand, he wants to encourage the mother to return as often as necessary in order to build up his practice while, on the other hand, he is attempting to help her develop independence. If he truly helps her to handle the many vexing problems of child rearing and minor illnesses, he will develop a pleasant practice with a limited number of frustrating telephone calls and few night visits. However, this is poor economics for the pediatrician starting out in practice. He would do better financially if he permitted the parents to have a little anxiety and encourage them to depend on him through frequent office visits. (Coddington, 1959:1008)

RESPONDING TO THE DISSATISFIED PEDIATRICIAN SYNDROME

The letters elicited a range of responses. Some pediatricians minimized the problem. They described the discontent as an isolated phenomenon, the experience of a relatively small number of practitioners who had erred in their choice of specialty and were personally unsuited for pediatric practice. What pediatricians needed above all else, the argument went, was a love of children. They needed to be able to find satisfaction in keeping their young charges well, and not merely in the high drama of curing rare, exotic diseases. For example, Borden Veeder, editor of the *Journal of Pediatrics* in the period through which many of these letters were published, offered the following editorial comment: "While it is unfortunate when a physician makes a wrong choice and as a result finds himself unhappy and discontented, the fault almost always lies in the individual and blame cannot be shifted to the particular field. . . . Look within thyself when things go wrong, is a wise maxim even if it is unpleasant to the ego" (Veeder, 1958:769). Lee F. Hill, president of the ABP, the specialty's licensing board, responded specifically to Tabrah's suggestion that interest in pediatrics might be waning and cited figures showing that there had been no significant decline in the number of specialty certificates granted by the board. He argued: "These figures clearly indicate sustained interest in pediatrics as a specialty and suggest that dissatisfaction with practice is on an individual basis" (Hill, 1957:747).

Others were less kind in their criticism. "Those who find pediatrics monotonous and boring," responded Wyman Cole (1959:642), the chair of the Section on Pediatrics at the annual meeting of the American Medical Association, "are practising with their eyes shut." He went on:

They are lacking in an awareness of what pediatrics is. They are miscast and should be in some other type of work. Of the thousands of time I have discussed with a young mother her perfectly normal baby, I have never once found it boring. She may have memorized Dr. Spock's excellent book from cover to cover, but she needs something more, the personal touch. It is gratifying to feel that you are giving this mother confidence and starting a new family off in the right direction. It is not as dramatic as cardiac catheterization, but it is more basic and in the long run more important. (Cole, 1959:642)

But there were also those who sympathized with the dissatisfied pediatricians and were concerned that the problem was much larger than a few personalities in the wrong specialty. They accused the pediatric leadership of trying to ignore the tell-tale signs of serious, underlying difficulties in the specialty and of burying their heads, ostrich-like, in the sand. Wineberg (1959:1008), a practising pediatrician from Waukegan, Illinois wrote:

> Pediatric practice consists of 85 to 90 percent of minor illness and well baby care. The remaining 10 to 15 percent often requires the highly skillful and specialized training for which pediatricians were prepared. When one becomes dissatisfied, the argument is that he has defects of personality, and after all, it is very wonderful to watch children grow and have patients invest so much faith in their doctor. Regardless of such rationalizations as these, if a man spends two years devoted to acquiring a highly specialized skill and then enters a practice which 90 percent of the time does not require this skill, then he has not really been trained for a specialty. . . . To admit that we are in a field which has less to offer than we havebeen taught is distressing. To continue to mislead fine young men into aspecialty that does not exist is more than unfortunate. (Wineberg, 1959: 1007–1008)

Moreover, there was evidence to support the claim of some of the letter writers that the dissatisfaction was widespread. A survey conducted by *Medical Economics* (1956) showed that pediatricians were medicine's most frustrated specialists and confirmed that many of them were, in fact, switching to other areas of medical practice. Ninety-five percent of the pediatricians surveyed were glad they had chosen medicine as a career, but only 63% were satisfied with their chosen specialty. They represented the lowest proportion of satisfied practitioners among all the specialists surveyed.

A 1960 national survey of 1227 pediatricians in private practice who had graduated after 1945 found that 64% of the respondents felt pediatric practice had not met their expectations. An open-ended question asking about what they considered to be "the principal problem(s) in the practice of pediatrics, both professionally and personally, today" (Aldrich and Spitz, 1960:71–72) elicited comments such as the following:

> I never realized that it would be so demanding of my time. It is practically a 24-hour daily job and seven days a week.
>
> The amount of referral work is much less than I expected.

More of a "general practice" in children than a specialty.

Like all newly practising pediatricians, I suppose I expected to see more "exotic" or at least more really problem cases than has been the case. I must concur with the opinion that minor problems constitute the great majority of my "sick-child" visits.

I see many more well patients for routine check up and immunizations than I did the first 15 years of practice.

The public's attitude toward the pediatrician is that toward a general practitioner and not toward a specialist.

The main professional problem in pediatrics is how to remain a well-informed child specialist when the nature of modern pediatric practice in terms of the kinds of problems one sees (well-baby care in office and respiratory infections at home) takes so much time that it is not possible to continue to grow and develop in this specialty as I believe we should.

I had anticipated practising pediatrics, not placating parents.

One commentator summarized the survey's findings by saying: "There is no need to cut butter with a razor. . . . What the questionnaire has done is to confirm what people have said in other contexts, that pediatricians apparently do have problems (Spitz, 1960:17).

These national survey results mirrored several smaller regional surveys such as a Washington state study (Deisher et al., 1960) that showed there was little correlation between the professional interests of pediatricians and the content of their practices. They had a low to moderate interest in the types of cases they mostly saw, including well-baby care, minor respiratory infections, vomiting, and diarrhea. The types of cases that most interested them, such as viral diseases, rheumatic fever, and prematurity, occurred infrequently, if at all.

More ominous to the specialty's leadership was the fact that pediatrics was losing its appeal among medical students. Samuel Levine (1960), president of the APS in 1960, acknowledged that for the first time in its history, pediatrics was having trouble attracting promising candidates. AMA directories showed that pediatrics, along with other low-status specialties such as anesthesiology, pathology, and psychiatry, had among the highest number of vacant residency positions. A survey conducted by the Association of Medical Colleges (Gee, 1960:37) among graduating seniors in 21 medical schools found that of the 103 seniors indicating a desire to specialize in pediatrics before their year of internship, only 56 were still interested in the specialty after their internship. The dissatisfied pediatrician syndrome was becoming a problem the specialty could not ignore.

Discussions about resolving the syndrome revolved first around pediatric training programs. The root of the dissatisfied pediatrician syndrome, some pediatricians suggested, lay in the education of primary care pediatricians and the expectations it created about the kind of medicine they could expect to practice once out of school. Their training focused on the high drama of life and death medicine, while private practice revolved around the more mundane aspects of prevention, health maintenance and routine care. In the words of yet another dissatisfied pediatrician: "while he had been trained to race at the Hialeah race track, he was now out pulling the chuck wagon like any old dray horse" (in Ambuel, 1959:1009–1010). Pediatricians were not trained for the primary care practices most would eventually find themselves in.

Pediatric academics came into the line of fire for being "unrealistic" and "out of touch with life outside the ivory tower" (Senn, 1956:614). They had not been "sufficiently sensitive to the changing nature of pediatrics in the modern American community" (Richmond, 1959:1177) and needed to learn how to train primary care pediatricians "not in their own image," but in the health care tasks and day-to-day problems they could actually expect to encounter once in practice. Once the discrepancy between training and practice was corrected, many felt, the problem of the dissatisfied pediatrician would disappear. Pediatricians would eventually learn to find satisfaction in their primary care careers.

But a number of pediatricians began to argue that as essential as it was to make training more reflective of primary care practice, educational reform on its own would not resolve the dissatisfied pediatrician syndrome. If the specialty wanted to secure its future, it needed to find new challenges and to redefine itself entirely. It needed to move into new areas of care that would give those practising primary care pediatrics a sense of purpose and professional satisfaction. The specialty needed a fundamental reorientation and that reorientation needed to be incorporated into pediatric education as well.

A NEW DIRECTION FOR PEDIATRICS?

As early as 1935, in an address to the Pediatric Section of the California Medical Association, Henry Stafford (1936) had warned that if pediatricians were going to survive the declines in mortality among children, they would have to be "on the alert" for new fields of endeavor. "Most of these fields," he wrote (1936:378), "deal with borderline problems, shades of difference between health and disease, conditions whereby the child is not invalided, but his social and individual efficiency is decreased." As some pediatricians sought new challenges they hoped would rejuvenate the specialty, they increasingly turned to such "borderline problems." They started to promote a new image of pediatrics, one that came to be called the "new pediatrics" (Talbot, 1960:913; White, 1955:537).

The new pediatrics focused not so much on the diseases of children as on children themselves and on their total well-being. "The goal of pediatrics," wrote Waldo Nelson (1955:112), a professor of pediatrics at Temple University School of Medicine, was "to assist the child to become an adult able to compete at a level approaching his optimal capacity and to assume his share of responsibility within the community." To fulfill that mandate, the specialty could not restrict itself merely to children's physical problems. Its scope of practice needed to incorporate anything that might threaten the development of children into healthy, happy, responsible and productive adults. The pediatrician's duty was to ensure children's complete physical, mental, emotional, psychological, and social growth and development. Defined in this way, Nelson (1955:112) insisted, pediatrics was "just coming of age rather than having fulfilled its mission." Grover Powers (1955:692), a contributing editor to *Pediatrics*, wrote:

> I believe that general child care . . . in all its possible ramifications may be developed in such manner as to offer a challenge to mind and personality as rewarding and satisfying to the physician who loves children as the drama of care restricted to the sick child.

Among the first proponents or crusaders for the new pediatrics were general pediatricians who were hired by departments of pediatrics through the 1950s to provide students with the experience in ambulatory pediatrics that department heads hoped would better prepare them for the harsh realities of private, primary care practice. Several of the experimental programs they established are described in the pediatric literature (Deisher, 1953a,b; Green and Senn, 1958; Green and Stark, 1957; Rose and Ross, 1960; Rogers, 1960; Senn, 1956; Solnit and Senn, 1954). Besides teaching, these general pediatricians ran outpatient clinics connected to teaching hospitals and eventually began to publish studies related to their teaching and patient care activities. As Halpern (1990:33) points out, once hired, these academics developed an interest in securing a place for their concerns among the specialty's scientific subspecialties.

But the new pediatrics also had the endorsement of many of pediatric's leaders who saw an expansion in the specialty's parameters as the only solution to the problem of the dissatisfied pediatrician. Samuel Levine (1960:653), president of the APS in 1960, stated in his presidential address: "If the role of the practising pediatrician is to promote child health and not just to cure or even prevent organic illness, then his task is far more challenging, exciting and important than it was even in the heyday of curative pediatrics." He encouraged the profession to respond to the disenchantment among pediatricians by adopting a new understanding of the pediatrician as a guardian of child health in its broadest possible terms:

> The young pediatrician today, if he engages in private practice, faces a real opportunity to promote all aspects of child life and health in his community—mental, emotional and social as well as just physical. If we can point out this challenge . . . and make the challenge sufficiently exciting and rewarding, pediatric practice, it seems to me, can face an era as golden as any we have known in the past. (Levine, 1960:656)

George Wheatley (1961a:836), president of the AAP in 1961, criticized those who suggested that the specialty abandon primary care, calling them unrealistic, defeatist, and unimaginative. The high consumer demand for pediatricians, he insisted, proved that the public wanted the profession to play a greater role in routine child care. Pediatricians had an obligation to respond to public needs. They also had an obligation to children that extended beyond their physical diseases. "The dimension to which we have given nearly all our attention so far," he wrote (1961a:837), "is the physical. . . . The pediatrician of tomorrow must be prepared to serve the 'whole' child." He urged progress "toward that ever-new concept of our specialty as yet unrealized—care of the 'whole' child."

There was a broad range of problems in child health care, the proponents of the new pediatrics argued, that still demanded understanding and solution. They pointed first to a long list of problem behaviors, or what were increasingly referred to as developmental, behavioral, emotional, or psychosocial problems—thumbsucking, stealing, stubbornness, tantrums, weepiness, destructiveness, biting, kicking, nervousness, being picked on, head banging, nail biting, nightmares, soiling, bullying, lying, school problems, trouble with authority, overweight, stealing, and truancy (Talbot, 1963:914). If pediatricians intervened early to treat these problems they could forestall more serious difficulties with juvenile delinquency and psychological maladjustment later in life.

> The babies whom we look after today will soon be the adult citizens of our Democracy. Even with our present very imperfect understanding of growth and adaptation we have really incontrovertible evidence that many influences which play their part in the early years of life have a profound effect on later behavior, happiness and even physical health of the individ-

ual. In view of these considerations it is difficult indeed to escape the conclusion that the pediatrician has *the moral obligation* to familiarize himself with these factors as well as he has familiarized himself with the doses of antibiotics or the amount of ACTH to give a rheumatic fever patient. In terms of the final crippling of the life of his patient, or making him a liability rather than an asset to our democratic society, it might even be more important to be able to recognize the dangers in a distorted mother-child relationship in infancy and know what to do about it. (Washburn, 1951:304; emphasis added)

Pediatricians could help chronically ill and handicapped children, and their families, by familiarizing themselves with the resources available to them, by helping them with problems of adjustment, and by fostering more accepting attitudes toward the handicapped in society. In the area of adoption, pediatricians could advise and counsel the natural mother, protecting her moral and legal rights and help her reach a decision she could comfortably live with the rest of her life, making sure the adoptive home was suitable for the child, exploring the motivations of families seeking to adopt, acting as an intermediary in arranging adoptions, and guiding adoptive parents through their unique difficulties. In relation to school health, pediatricians could do more to foster good student–teacher relations and were uniquely situated to interpret and correct problems the child might have in school. With accidents topping the list of major childhood killers since 1950, pediatricians could look for more effective ways to help parents prevent poisonings, burns, home accidents, and bicycle and pedestrian accidents (Fischer, 1957).

An important dimension of the new pediatrics was "anticipatory guidance," which one pediatrician (Hill, 1960:301) defined as "the anticipation for parents and interpretation to them of expected normal patterns of behavior in children as they occur in various age groups." If pediatricians were going to fulfill their obligations to children, they would have to pay more attention to their parents and to encourage a rich and rewarding parental experience. Rather than waiting for parents to raise questions about child rearing spontaneously, they should raise these subjects themselves and facilitate discussions of any potential problem. In fact, some suggested that parents should leave the child at home and meet with the pediatrician alone for such guidance (Crook, in Deisher, 1960:21).

In addressing the "unmet" problems of children, pediatricians were also exhorted to look beyond the traditional age group of pediatrics. An area the specialty had barely begun to exploit, some specialty leaders told them, was the health problems of children over 12 years of age. After all, adolescence was a natural extension of childhood, a continuation of the growth and development process that was the basis of pediatric practice. The pediatrician's task was not complete until children had progressed safely through their adolescent years. Pediatricians were encouraged to make a "special effort to understand the puzzling problems and potential of adolescence" (Levine, 1960:655). George Wheatley (1961b:160) observed:

> This is a twilight zone in medical practice, upon which more light needs to be shed. I hope that pediatricians will take the initiative to study the needs of this group. The important point is that these children should be encouraged to visit pediatricians and more pediatricians should be equipping themselves to understand and cope with teen-age health problems.

The adjustments to a rapidly changing body and development of secondary sex characteristics, the new gynecological concerns of girls becoming young women, acne, the preoccupation with peer standards, with fitting in and appearing "normal," the struggle with adult responsibilities, and the propensity for strenuous activity and sports injuries that often resulted, were just some of the unique health problems faced by adolescents that had yet to be addressed (Gallagher, 1954, 1982). The teen years were also seen to be a critical time for anticipatory guidance. The adolescent's need for independence and parents' reluctance to "loosen the apron strings" often made relations between them tense. Sexual maturation and the responsibilities that accompany it were often an area of conflict between parents and children. Pediatricians, if they were willing to take on these problems on, could guide parent, as well as child, through adolescence (Hill, 1960:302).

RESISTING THE REORIENTATION

The commitment to the new pediatrics among some in pediatrics' academic elite was reflected not only in the hiring of general pediatricians to prepare students for primary care, but in the establishment of fellowship programs in the new pediatrics. Through the 1960s fellowships were created in areas such as behavioral sciences and psychiatry, child development, community pediatrics, care of handicapped children and mental retardation, and adolescent medicine. But by 1969, there were only 16 such fellowships, and they constituted only 13% of all pediatric fellowships available (Friedman, 1970:173), indicating that the attitude toward the new pediatrics was still uncertain.

As the specialty began to move, however tentatively, in the direction of the new pediatrics, educators who opposed the redefinition and expansion of pediatrics became more vocal. They insisted that the new pediatrics took the specialty too far afield of its traditional medical mission—to treat and prevent physical diseases—and that the image and stature of pediatrics as an academic specialty would suffer as a result. They sympathized with the problems of practising pediatricians but were not willing to sacrifice their own interests to give practitioners a new lease on life. Pediatrics was already having trouble attracting high caliber students to its programs. Opponents were convinced that the further the specialty moved in the direction of the new pediatrics, the more aggravated the recruitment problem would become. Robert E. Cook, the director of the Pediatrics Department at Johns Hopkins University School of Medicine, argued that to solve the problem of the dissatisfied pediatrician by teaching the new pediatrics would create only another problem—the dissatisfied student. "To substitute in the limited hours we have much more of the behavioral approach," he maintained (in Korsch, 1960:42), "would mean . . . loss of interest for pediatrics by those students for whom it has some appeal."

The evidence suggests that Cook was right. Those programs that experimented with a more comprehensive and behaviorally oriented pediatrics found that students resented spending time on anything not directly relevant to the treatment and prevention of disease. At the University of Colorado, where one such program had been set up, students complained they felt "cheated" with respect to medical knowledge compared to students in traditional pediatric programs. "They thought they weren't seeing enough sick patients and were seeing far too many patients who really didn't have anything wrong with them, from whom they weren't learning anything" (Hammond, in Spitz, 1960:27).

The developers of a program in the new pediatrics at Yale University (Green and Senn, 1958:490) conceded that the prototype of the pediatrician in the minds of most students was still "one who is concerned with physical disease alone." The residents applied a double standard to organic and nonorganic aspects of a medical problem. They were preoccupied with the possibility of overlooking organic pathology, but less concerned about missing important psychosocial factors. Many did not believe that knowledge about the psychosocial aspects of pediatrics would be important in their practice or research careers. Green and Senn (1958) described this attitude as a "major deterrent" to the full integration of the new pediatrics into their program.

The reservations of some within the academic community were expressed most clearly by Charles D. May (1960), a professor at the Columbia University College of Physicians and Surgeons. May insisted that pediatricians had no business embracing the emotional and behavioral problems of children. They were transgressing not only the limits of their technical competence, but the bounds of their legal licenses as well.

According to May, pediatricians did have a unique contribution to make to the welfare of children, but as doctors, not counselors. In the area of behavioral development they had little to offer beyond their love of children. However, a sound specialty, he went on to argue, "cannot be based on the sentimental appeal of a fondness of children" (May, 1960:662). He warned:

> the pediatrician, as a member of the medical profession, must not allow his ambition to outstrip his abilities, lest he take on greater responsibilities than he can manage or find to his liking. . . . The unique role of most pediatricians for the foreseeable future will be as physicians, rather than as psychologists or general counselors. They should not delude themselves by supposing they can become a priestly class of counselors on all things. Let those who would choose to be primarily counselors set themselves apart, or enter the ranks of other professions. (May, 1960:662–663)

For May, pediatricians' very status as part of the medical profession was at stake: "Unless limits are set, the primary task of physical care will be diluted and dislocated beyond recognition and the pediatrician may no longer be considered a physician" (May, 1960:663). May pleaded with pediatricians to put the needs of the specialty ahead of those of dissatisfied primary care pediatricians. "The problems facing pediatrics," he concluded (May, 1960:662), were to "do something to elevate the status and appeal of the practice of pediatrics to that of a genuine and significant specialty and to make certain that the prestige and validity of academic pediatrics are unquestioned, *regardless of how the domestic care of children may be accomplished.*"

May recommended that the profession sharply curtail the number of residencies for specialty training in pediatrics so that "no more pediatricians are produced than can find place as genuine specialists" (May, 1960:666). He also suggested that pediatricians curtail any research activities in the area of children's behavioral problems. Otherwise, he predicted, contributions from the field of pediatrics "will be characterized by superficiality and receive less serious respect from investigators in other branches in medical science" (May, 1960:668).

May's sentiments were echoed a year later by L. Emmett Holt, Jr., in his presidential address to the APS. He described eloquently and sympathetically the plight of the primary care pediatrician: "They were intrigued by medicine; they wanted to be doctors; they wanted to treat sick children, and they were trained to do just that. Now they find that the sick child is the exceptional one they are asked to see" (Holt, 1961:675). But he expressly rejected the new pediatrics as a response to the problem. Instead, the "wonder drug" that Holt recommended for dissatisfied pediatricians was foreign service. American pediatricians were "painting lilies," "struggling with refinements," and becoming "more and more engrossed in minutiae," while children overseas were dying of smallpox and starvation. The solution was obvious: "We must take our tools abroad and apply them to our neighbor's problems" (Holt, 1961:676).

There was resistance among practicing pediatricians as well. Many did not want to assume responsibility for children's social and behavioral problems because they did not see these as part of their professional task. They felt that pediatrics was venturing into areas in which it did not really belong and in which pediatricians had no expertise. "Has the practising pediatrician completely mined the medical aspects of his practice," complained Herbert Harned (1959:860), a practitioner in Chapel Hill, North Carolina, "so that he must now turn to the paramedical?" Harned acknowledged the range of needs in the area of children's social and emotional development. But he questioned the ability of pediatricians to make any real contribution in these areas:

> Should the pediatrician whose entire medical background (and oftentimes temperament) may not suit him for giving expert advice in schooling problems, adoption procedures and problems of social adjustment be the one to till this vacuum? Cannot many of these questions be more effectively answered by social workers, guidance counselors, ministers, lawyers and other personnel? (Harned, 1959:860)

Practitioners complained they were "coerced" into areas of practice that exceeded both their training and inclinations. One pediatrician pointed out: "In choosing pediatrics as a career one expresses a real concern for young people but not necessarily for the totality of their life and existence" (Work, 1970:173).

When the pediatric literature began to reflect the interests of some pediatricians in the nonmedical problems of children, reactions were sometimes strong and negative. For example, when the journal *Pediatrics* published research on young male prostitutes with an accompanying editorial entitled "Bisexuality Gone Astray," which elaborated on problems of sexual identity and sexual development among adolescents, one pediatrician (Hick, 1970:153) suggested that it was pediatrics that was going astray. He advised the journal to appoint a critic for its editorial board—someone to more carefully screen its content for relevance and appropriateness and to save it from "future embarrassment in its laudable effort to broaden the pediatrician's role in society." Another paper in *Pediatrics* on school problems elicited this response in a letter to the editor: "A nonmedical subspecialty problem is not a remedy for the 'pediatric disenchantment syndrome'" (Schmitt, 1969:772). The correspondent went on to argue that the school is the proper place to solve school problems, not the pediatrician's office; and the school psychologist is the proper person to handle such problems, not the pediatrician.

The 1950s and 1960s, then, were a period of serious soul-searching for pediatrics as various segments of the specialty debated the causes of the widespread disaffection among primary care practitioners, analyzed the specialty's difficulties, proposed solutions, and tried to forge a direction for the future. While they debated, more ominous threats loomed.

Chapter 4

The Supply Crisis

INTRODUCTION

The dissatisfied pediatrician syndrome of the 1950s and 1960s was primarily a crisis of purpose. An ever-growing number of pediatricians were not satisfied with primary care pediatrics. By the 1970s the specialty found itself dealing with a different crisis. New groups of child health care workers were emerging—pediatric nurse practitioners and family practitioners. Unlike many pediatricians these groups were eager to minister to the routine health care needs of children. Birth rates, in the meantime, were falling, which meant that while the number of child health care professionals was on the rise, the number of children requiring their services was on a decline.

These developments added a new dimension to pediatrics' problems. In addition to its crisis of purpose, the specialty now faced a supply crisis. The question was no longer simply whether primary care pediatricians could find satisfaction in their work, but whether there was going to be work for them in child health care. The supply crisis gave a greater urgency to the search for a new mission that would give primary care pediatricians a sense of professional fulfillment and at the same time secure a place for them in child health care. In this chapter I document the rise of the supply crisis and describe the interprofessional rivalries that it created between pediatricians and their competitors in child health care.

CHANGING TRENDS

Much of the overwork that pediatricians complained about through the 1950s and 1960s resulted from the surge in the number of births after World War II—the baby boom. But after 1957 the boom leveled off and both the birth rate, which represents births per thousand population,

61

and the actual number of live births began to decline (see Table 3.1). The birth rate fell 6% from 25.3 per 1000 population in 1957 to 23.7 in 1060, another 22% to 18.4% in 1970, and a further 14% to 15.9 in 1980. The number of live births fell from 4.3 million in 1957 to 4.2 in 1960, 3.7 in 1970, and 3.6 in 1980.

Several interrelated trends contributed to the declines, the most significant of which was the shift toward more effective means of contraception, especially the birth control pill. Other factors included the transformation in women's roles that the women's liberation movement precipitated, changing social mores about reproduction and ideal family size, concern about world population growth, and the 1970 Supreme Court decision to legalize abortion.

The pill was developed in the late 1950s and approved for sale by the Federal Drug Administration in 1960 (Reed, 1978:365). It rapidly became the most popular method of contraception, despite the debate about possible side effects. A national fertility study showed that by 1970 the pill accounted for 34% of all contraceptive practices. The next most common method was sterilization at 16%. The pill was especially popular among women under 35 years of age. In 1970, 49% in this age group who practiced contraception used the pill, compared with 21% of women over 35 years of age (Westoff and Ryder, 1977:21).

The absolute number of children below 5 years of age dropped from 20.3 million in 1960 to 17.2 million in 1970, and then in subsequent age categories. The total number of children under 20 years of age rose until 1970 because it continued to include the baby boom cohorts. In 1960 there were 69 million individuals under 20 years of age; in 1965 there were 76.7 million, and in 1970 there were 77.1 million. In 1975, however, the figure dropped to 74.4 million, and in 1980 to 72.5 million (see Table 4.1 for the actual and projected total number of children and breakdowns by age). The market for pediatric services was clearly shrinking.

The declines in the birth rate were greatest in precisely those groups that were at the highest risk for premature and low-birth-weight babies, conditions associated with illnesses during childhood. These groups included women with several children, older women, and unwed mothers. The percentage of births to women with five or more children decreased 75% from 17 in 1960 to 5 in 1973. Conversely, the percentage of first-born babies increased 14% from 26 in 1960 to 41 in 1973 (Table 4.2). In the same years, the number of births to women 30 years of age and over decreased 55% from 1.14 million to 518,856 (Table 4.2). The legalization of abortion accounted for much of the reductions in both the number and percentage of births to unwed mothers. Between 1970, the year abortion became legal, and 1971, the number of legal abortions in the United Sates jumped from 200,000 to 500,000. Three-fifths of all those

Table 4.1. Number of Children and Adolescents by Age[a] and Year

	Age Ranges				
Year	0–4	5–9	10–14	15–19	Total
1960	20.3	18.7	16.8	13.2	69.0
1965	20.2	20.5	18.9	17.1	76.7
1970	17.2	20.0	20.8	19.1	77.1
1975	16.2	17.4	20.0	20.8	74.4
1980	16.5	16.6	18.2	21.2	72.5
1985	18.5	16.6	16.8	18.4	70.3
1990[b]	19.2	18.6	16.8	17.0	71.6
1995[b]	18.6	19.3	18.8	17.0	73.7
2000[b]	17.6	18.8	19.5	18.9	74.8

[a] In millions.
[b] Projected.
Sources: AMA Council on Long Range Planning and Development (1987:242); Gorwitz and Smith (1975:595).

who received abortions were under 25 years of age and two-thirds of them were unmarried (Sklar and Berkov, 1974:909).

Predictably, the number of low-birth-weight babies fell. In 1960, 23,008 babies weighed less than 1000 grams at birth. In 1973, there were 16,761, a drop of 27%; those weighing 2500 grams or less at birth de-

Table 4.2. Selected Data on Live Births: 1960–1973

	1960	1973	Percentage Change
Total	4,257,850	3,144,198	−26.2
By Birth Order			
1	1,090,152	1,319,126	+21.0
2	1,022,356	985,726	−3.9
3	797,402	441,404	−44.7
4	511,308	183,925	−64.0
5>	715,234	176,693	−75.3
By Age of Mother			
Under 15	6,780	12,642	+46.4
15–19	586,966	582,238	−0.8
20–24	1,426,912	1,093,676	−23.4
25–29	1,092,816	936,786	−14.3
30–34	687,722	375,500	−45.4
35–39	359,908	115,409	−67.9
40–44	91,564	26,319	−71.3
45–49	5,042	1,628	−67.7
50>	140	—	−100.0

Source: U.S. National Center for Health Statistics (1960: 2–10, 2–22; 1978: 1–70, 1–73, 1–226).

creased 28% from 327,484 to 236,270 in 1973 (Table 4.2). The mortality in all childhood age groups also fell after 1950. The infant mortality rate declined from 29.2 in 1950 to 26 in 1960, 20 in 1970, and 12.6 in 1980, a 57% drop over thirty years. There was another 57% drop in mortality among children between 1 and 4 years of age, from 1.4 in 1960 to 0.6 in 1980. For children between 5 and 14 years of age, there was a 50% drop from 0.6 in 1950 to 0.3 in 1980 (see Table 2.3).

NEW CHILD HEALTH CARE PROVIDERS

While the number of children declined, the number of health care providers for children increased dramatically. The increase was part of a large expansion in medical personnel in the United States through the 1960s and 1970s. The 1960s had generated a heated debated about the inadequacies of the American health care system. Though science had made tremendous strides in conquering illness, critics argued, there were many who were not benefiting from the new knowledge. Minorities, the poor, and those living in inner-city or in rural areas were particularly disadvantaged. Construed largely as a labor supply problem—too few doctors, especially at the primary care level—the response was a massive government-sponsored effort to improve access to health care.

Federal expenditure in health manpower programs grew astronomically from $65 million in 1963 to $536 million in 1973 and $1.7 billion in 1977 (*Journal of the AMA*, 1980). The number of medical schools increased from 86 in 1960 to 126 in 1980 (Table 4.3). Established medical schools expanded and increased their capacity, particularly through the 1970s. The total enrollment in medical schools more than doubled between 1960 and 1980 from 30,288 to 64,195; so too did the number of graduates, from 6994 in 1960 to 15,135 in 1980. The number of doctors rose from 274,800 in 1960 to 467,700 in 1980 (Table 4.4).

Pediatrics, as a primary care specialty, profited from the increased funding. The number of pediatricians increased from 14,273 in 1964 to 23,959 in 1977 (AAP, 1980:20; Gorwitz and Smith, 1975:595). But so too did other groups, particularly paramedical workers. The Federal government had established training programs for new types of allied health care workers or "physician extenders." As the term "physician extend er" suggests, such programs increased the productivity and efficiency of doctors by training other groups to do work that did not require a doctor's skills.

In pediatrics there were several such categories of workers including pediatric aides, pediatric assistants, and child health associates. Pediatric

Table 4.3. Expansion of Medical Education: Number of Medical Schools, Students, and Graduates

Year	Number of Schools	Total Enrollment	Graduates
1950–1951	79	26186	6135
1955–1956	82	28639	6845
1956–1957	85	29130	6796
1957–1958	85	29473	6861
1958–1959	85	29614	6860
1959–1960	85	30084	7081
1960–1961	86	30288	6994
1961–1962	87	31078	7168
1962–1963	87	31491	7264
1963–1964	87	32001	7336
1964–1965	88	32428	7409
1965–1966	88	32835	7574
1966–1967	89	33423	7743
1967–1968	94	34538	7973
1968–1969	99	35833	8059
1969–1970	101	37669	8367
1970–1971	103	40487	8974
1971–1972	108	43650	9551
1972–1973	112	47546	10391
1973–1974	114	50886	11613
1974–1975	114	54074	12714
1975–1976	114	56244	13561
1976–1977	116	58266	13607
1977–1978	122	60456	14393
1978–1979	125	62754	14966
1979–1980	126	64195	15135
1980–1981	126	65497	15667
1981–1982	126	66485	15985
1982–1983	127	66886	15824
1983–1984	127	67443	16327
1984–1985	127	67090	16347

Source: Journal of the AMA (1980–2813; 1985:1568).

aides were typically high school graduates with on-the-job training that allowed them to undertake routine, nonskilled tasks, perform clerical duties, and assist pediatricians. Pediatric assistants completed a special 2-year college program that emphasized technical skills. But in the performance of their duties, pediatric assistants did not assume responsibility for their decisions. Child health associates received more extensive training. Their program required 2 years of general undergraduate training as a prerequisite and then 3 years of special college training, including one internship year. Child health associates could take a direct role in patient care and make independent decisions, but

Table 4.4. Total Number of Doctors (in Thousands)

Year	Total Number Doctors	Year	Total Number Doctors
1950	203.4	1970	334.0
1951	205.5	1971	335.8
1952	207.9	1972	344.8
1953	210.9	1973	371.4
1954	214.2	1974	379.7
1955	218.1	1975	393.7
1956		1976	409.4
1957	226.6	1977	421.3
1958		1978	437.5
1959	236.8	1979	454.6
1960	274.8	1980	467.7
1961		1981	485.1
1962	270.1	1982	502.0
1963	289.1	1983	519.5
1964	297.1		
1965	305.1		
1966	313.6		
1967	322.0		
1968	330.7		
1969	338.9		

Sources: U.S. Bureau of the Census (1975); Statistical Abstracts 1970–1983.

only underthe supervision of a doctor (Ott, 1975:42–5). But the largest single allied health care group in pediatrics was the pediatric nurse practitioner (PNP).

Pediatric Nurse Practitioners (PNPs)

The crisis in health care delivery during the 1960s coincided with a desire among some nurses to redefine their traditional role and expand their scope of practice to include medical as well as nursing services (Schwartz, de Wolf, and Skipper, 1987). These nurses felt that they could perform many of the routine tasks usually reserved for doctors such as conducting physical examinations, formulating treatment plans, and managing patient care. Beyond easing the health care burden and presenting nurses with new challenges, nurses saw an expansion of their role into medical services as a way to enhance the status of their occupation from a subservient "handmaiden" (Backup and Molinaro, 1984:219) of medicine to that of a true profession.

Not all nurses wanted to take on medical functions. To some such a move represented not the expansion, but an abdication of the nursing role. Nursing was about promoting health, not seeking and controlling pathology, they insisted, and by providing medical services nurses were crossing the line that had always separated nurses from doctors:

> Persons who choose to leave nursing to become physicians' assistants, pediatric associates and the like, must find their identity in the new field they have chosen. They are no longer entitled to an identity as nurses. (Rogers, 1972:45)

Undeterred, those with greater ambitions for their profession created a new category—the nurse practitioner.

The nurse practitioner movement could not have succeeded without medical sponsorship. Pediatricians were the first group within medicine to help them. Though the nurse practitioner movement eventually expanded into other areas—obstetrics and gynecology, perinatal medicine, geriatrics, psychiatry, emergency medicine—it gained its first foothold in pediatrics. On the basis of its successes there the movement was able to grow.

Why were pediatricians so obliging to a group that wanted to take over aspects of the pediatrician's function? Under different circumstances, pediatricians might have perceived the redefinition of the nurse's role as an encroachment into their professional preserve. But caught in the grips of the dissatisfied pediatrician syndrome, pediatricians saw the nurse practitioner as a potential solution to the specialty's problems. By taking over the more routine, day-to-day activities of pediatric primary care pediatricians thought nurse practitioners might be able to relieve them of the boredom and monotony that was making medical practice so unfulfilling for them. Moreover, nurse practitioners were willing to work in those areas—inner-cities and rural regions—that pediatricians tended to find unattractive. Their mutual interests thus aligned, pediatricians and nurses came together to create the first nurse practitioner programs in the country.

In 1964, Henry Silver, a pediatrician, and Loretta Ford, a public health nurse, organized a 4-month PNP program at the University of Colorado's School of Nursing. The program provided registered nurses with intensive training in pediatric theory and practice (Silver, Ford, and Stearly, 1967) so that they could assume "the 89 to 90 percent of pediatric practice which is concerned with well children and with relatively mild disease states" (Breslau, 1982:388–389). They were taught how to complete a pediatric history, perform a comprehensive basic physical examination, carry out immunizations, determine the developmental status of the child, evaluate hearing, speech, and vision, perform certain basic tests, evaluate and manage the common medical problems of childhood, counsel parents, assist in the management of emergencies, care for newborn infants, make home visits, and handle telephone calls. The University of Colorado program served as a model for others. With government support, the number of PNP programs grew to over 50 by 1973 (Bullough, Sultz, Henry, and Fiedler, 1984:194). By 1977, there were more than 4000 graduates of such programs (Breslau, 1982:389). PNPs worked either in pediatricians' offices or in medical clinics in low-income, urban, and rural areas. Legally, they were required to work under the supervision of doctors. But in many clinics, particularly in ghettoes or outlying areas, medical supervision meant only an occasional visit from a pediatrician. In effect then, some PNPs were practising independently or semi-independently.

Pediatric sponsorship of PNPs amounted to more than assisting nurses to set up and run the first PNP programs and hiring the graduates of such programs. Pediatricians were instrumental in selling the concept of "the nurse practitioner" to the rest of the medical profession. They helped demonstrate that nurse practitioners could indeed perform medical tasks effectively and efficiently, that patients were willing to accept nurses in this new role, and perhaps, most importantly, that the hiring of nurse practitioners could be cost-effective.

Through the 1960s and 1970s the medical literature demonstrated how effectively PNPs were functioning as child health care providers. In a child health clinic in Denver, Colorado, in which 54% of all visits were for well-child care and 46% for illnesses and injuries, PNPs cared for 82% of the children on their own, referring only 18% to a doctor (Silver, 1968:488). In another Denver child health clinic, the physical examinations that PNPs conducted yielded assessments that were very close to those of pediatricians. In 240 out of 278 (86%) cases, there was complete agreement between PNPs and pediatricians in their assessments. In 39 (14%) cases, there was a difference but in only two cases (0.7%) was that difference significant (Duncan, Smith, and Silver, 1971). In a Pittsburgh health center situated in a low-income housing project, the performance of PNPs rated highly in the area of infant health supervision, as measured by the number of well-child visits, the health status of infants at 1 year of age, and comparison with children in an upper socioeconomic private pediatric practice (Chappell and Drogos, 1972). Moreover, PNPs lowered the failed appointment rate from 60% at the beginning of the study to 20%. At St. Louis University, PNPs achieved scores on written examinations comparable to those of pediatric residents and better than those of senior medical students (DeCastro and Rolfe, 1974).

In fact, one study (Stehbens and Lauer, 1972) showed that PNPs functioned competently not only in primary care, but in specialized areas of pediatrics as well. When the demand for pediatric cardiology consultations in Iowa exceeded the capacity of a state-sponsored clinic to provide these services, the clinic decided to employ three PNPs. Assessments of their performance showed that their scores on written tests of factual knowledge were comparable to those of medical students. In cardiological examinations, the PNPs achieved a 93% agreement rate with pediatric cardiologists. They were better than the cardiologists at picking up other medical problems. Out of 307 cardiac examinations, the PNPs identified 69 cases of mental retardation, hearing impairment, congenital abnormalities, allergies, and acute respiratory infections. The pediatric cardiologists recorded only 14 problems.

The studies established as well that the public accepted an expanded role for pediatric nurses (Patterson, Bergman, and Wedgewood, 1969). Those who study professions (Bucher, 1980:26) have explained why public acceptance is so critical to the creation of a new occupational category in medicine and why sponsoring professions pay so much attention to how they present these groups to their clientele. Clients, they point out, expect and have always received certain services from doctors. They may reject the notion of receiving them from anyone else, thus undermining efforts to integrate the new workers. This explains why the literature of sponsoring groups is preoccupied with the acceptance of such workers. Pediatricians had particular cause for concern because the group to which they were now delegating their work—the nurse—was one with which patients were already familiar and that they viewed in stereotypical ways.

Pediatric studies, however, showed that there was no need for pediatricians to worry about resistance from clients. Schiff, Fraser, and Walters (1969) observed that in their suburban pediatric practice, mothers frequently began dressing their children and preparing to leave the office even before the pediatrician had the opportunity to confirm the PNPs assessment. They also observed that parents were making appointments directly with the PNP. A Denver pediatrician, Lewis Day, found in his study that 94% of his patients were happy with the services they received from his PNP, Rosemarie Egli; 57% stated that the joint care provided by Day and Egli was better than the care they received from Day alone.

I feel that the nurse practitioner is very beneficial to Dr. Day and to the community.

I feel Miss Egli is the greatest thing to happen to pediatrics. Nurse practitioners should surely become a trend in the future.

I believe this is a wonderful innovation. I wholeheartedly endorse this program and feel everyone would benefit from such excellent care. (Day, Egli, and Silver, 1970:207)

Patients liked the accessibility and approachability of PNPs and liked being able to deal with more than one health care professional:

The main point I like is calling and getting questions answered that I normally wouldn't have bothered Dr. Day with.

I think that the two of them together make my visit shorter and much more informative than I have experienced with any other doctor.

When seeing two people it gives you a chance to think of all your questions that you would ordinarily forget and later wish you had remembered to ask.

As parents we receive more information than formerly.

I think the child gets a more thorough examination, and between the two of them they are less apt to miss something that might be wrong. (Day et al., 1970:207)

Stehbens and Lauer (1972) used a more sophisticated measure of patient satisfaction that included completeness of the examination, time spent with the patient, explanations provided, opportunity to ask questions, and perceived competence. The study found that PNPs scored higher than pediatric cardiologists on *all* measures of patient satisfaction.

Finally, the studies established that PNPs were not only affordable, but profitable for pediatric practices. Schiff et al. (1969) showed that their PNP increased the number of patients in their group practice by 18.8%. She reduced the average time that pediatricians spent with each patient from 14 to 4 minutes. Yankauer, Connelly, and Feldman (1972) calculated that while it cost $3197 to educate a PNP in the program at the Bunker Hill Health Center in the Massachusetts General Hospital, the average PNP saw 65 children per week and earned $9100 per year. The net income generating potential of PNPs over and above their salary averaged $2500 per nurse, per year. Fourteen of the 26 PNPs in the study were capable of generating $3000 per year over and above their salaries (Yankauer et al., 1972:878).

PNPs did not win the approval of all pediatricians. Some pediatricians were bothered by the idea of nurses taking over "doctor's work." William G. Crook, a practitioner in Jackson, Tennessee, commended PNPs for the care they provided in rural and ghetto areas where access to proper medical care was limited. "I can understand," he wrote (1969:934), "that a nurse practitioner working independently, . . . supervised only at a distance by a pediatrician is better for the people of such an area than having no health worker at all." But the practice set a dangerous precedent, he argued. What rationale would there be for increasing or even maintaining the current number of pediatricians, if PNPs, in a relatively short period of time and at greatly reduced cost, could receive the training necessary to provide basic child health care:

> I fear that with our pediatric manpower shortage being what it is, the cost of providing health manpower so great, the federal government and others might seize on the nurse practitioner program as the way to get the job done at a low cost. . . .
>
> As a practising pediatrician, perhaps like all human beings I am threatened by change. Perhaps I am needlessly threatened; nevertheless, I believe that if training programs are set up for pediatric nurse assistants and other associates who will then enter upon independent or semi-independent practice, the trouble lies ahead. (Crook, 1969:933–934)

Glenn Austin, a practitioner in Los Altos, California, expressed similar reservations:

> The pediatrician is being told, in essence, that he is wasting 80 percent of his time on trivia that can be handled well by a nurse with a bit of pediatric training. Let us cease the patchwork PNP approach and instead improve pediatric residencies. . . . American children deserve the best in quality care, not poorly conceived and hastily trained part-time substitutes. (Austin, 1975:620)

But these reservation did not reflect the view of organized pediatrics. In 1970, the AAP officially endorsed the PNP concept. So too did a majority of the organization's members. A survey (Yankauer et al., 1970) found that 63% supported the training of PNPs and would be willing to hire one in their own practice. This figure, the authors of the study point out, actually underestimated the degree of acceptance since there were probably many among the remaining 34% who said they would not hire a PNP because they already had one on staff.

Family Practitioners

Another group that benefited from government support for primacy care providers was the budding specialty of family practice, which had its roots in general practice. General practice experienced a steady decline over the first half of the twentieth century. There were several factors working against general practice. First, the more attractive the specialties became over the course of the twentieth century, both in terms of prestige and income, the less able general practice was to compete. Second, the composition of medical school admission committees worked against the selection of students committed to general practice. The committees were comprised of scientifically oriented specialists who were biased toward candidates expressing an interest in specialty training and research. Third, medical school culture taught students to value the rare and interesting problems over more common clinical problems that might fill a career in general practice. Even students who entered medical school wanting a career in general practice often changed their minds by the time they graduated.

As the number of specialists increased, the number of general practitioners declined. In 1900, there was one general practitioner for every 600 people. By the late 1960s, there was one for every 3000 people. The ratio of general practitioners to specialists completely reversed itself from 4:1 in 1930 to approximately 1:4 in 1970 (Geyman, 1985:4). Many health care analysts predicted the eventual elimination of general practitioners except in isolated, outlying areas, and the commensurate growth of primary care specialties like pediatrics, internal medicine, and obstetrics and gynecology.

In some ways the dilemma of general practitioners was analogous to that of pediatricians. Both groups feared their imminent decline and possible disappearance as a distinct professional group. Both were eager to find a way to rejuvenate themselves. However, in one important respect their circumstances were different. Most pediatricians saw the specialty's original mandate as being largely fulfilled, and felt that what the specialty needed was a new direction and a new mission. General practitioners, on the other hand, remained convinced that there was still a place for the generalist in medicine. They sought not a new mission but a way to reassert the value of their original mission.

Ironically, while general practitioners remained strongly "generalist," to advance their generalist interests, they sought to become a specialty. On the face of it, the designation of general medicine as a specialty appears to be a contradiction in terms. But general practitioners believed that with the allure of specialism, the structure of American medical education, and especially the organization of medical schools into specialty departments, the only way to compete with other specialties for curriculum time, resources, and recruits was to become a specialty.

In 1947, general practitioners created an independent professional association—the American Academy of General Practitioners (AAGP)—modeled on the many existing specialty groups. The AAGP was in part the product of the growing fear of annihilation, but more immediately a reaction to general practitioners' negative wartime experiences. During World War II, general practitioners had suffered what they felt to be humiliating treatment within the military, receiving lower ranks and salaries, and fewer privileges than board-certified specialists. They were often sent to the front, while specialists received field hospital assignments (AAP, 1950:515; Stevens, 1971:277–280). They came out of the war angry and determined to protect their interests.

Through the 1950s, the AAGP organized hospital residency programs in general medicine. But the residencies were unpopular and attracted few students. There were neither financial, nor academic incentives to enroll. Those students that started the program often left after 1 year, a move that even the advocates of general medicine could understand. As one of them (Silver, 1963:188) put it: "no sensible student wants to spend three or four years becoming a general practitioner in order to work harder, earn less [than a specialist] and be banned from the hospital." Those who completed their residency were no further ahead than general practitioners who started practising right after their internships.

In the 1960s, the AAGP changed its strategy. Capitalizing on the growing dissatisfaction with the fragmentation in specialty care and concerned about the lack of primary care doctors, the AAGP began promoting a different image of the generalist in medicine—the "family practitioner." Family practice shared with general practice the qualities that people still valued and wanted in a doctor—a concern for the patient as an individual, accessibility, and the personal touch. But family practice was not merely general practice with a new name. In contrast to the traditional general practitioner and specialists who offered episodic, therapeutic care for a sick individual, the family practitioner offered coordinated, continuous, comprehensive care to all family members. The family, and not the individual, was the unit of care. And unlike general practitioners who had the image of well-meaning but antiquated anachronisms in the age of modern medicine, family practitioners would be trained to apply the latest scientific advances to total family health. To reflect its new orientation, the AAGP changed its name in 1971 to the American Academy of Family Practice (AAFP).

Family practice received a major boost as a new specialty in 1966 with the release of three major national reports on health care and medical education. The first was the report of the National Commission on Community Health Services (Folsom, 1966); the second was produced by the Citizens' Commission on Graduate Medical Education (Millis, 1966); the third was the report of the Ad Hoc Committee on Education for Family Practice of the Council on Medical Education (Willard, 1966). All three reports clearly identified the need for better comprehensive care at the primary level and strongly recommended that medical schools make a greater effort to prepare doctors for this role.

The AMA responded by granting family practice specialty status. In February 1969, the American Board of Family Practice (ABFP) joined the list of specialty boards in medicine. The Board was comprised of five representatives of the AAGP, five representatives of the AMA Section on General Practice, and one representative each from the specialties of internal medicine, pediatrics, surgery, psychiatry/neurology, and obstetrics/gynecology. Like other specialty boards, it did not have the power to restrict practice in the area of family medicine. But it could certify those who met the Board's requirements, including a 3 year family practice residency, and gave family practice official specialty status. In a gesture that could not more graphically illustrate the process of professional transformation that generalists were undergoing, the ABFP chose as its insignia the legendary phoenix, who sets itself ablaze only to arise, rejuvenated, from its own ashes.

The Federal government responded to the Folsom, Millis, and Willard reports with generous funding for family practice programs. In 1971, Congress passed the Comprehensive Health Manpower Training Act, a section of which specifically encouraged the development, expansion, and upgrading of residency programs in family practice. Between 1971 and 1977, the government provided over 33.5 million dollars for family practice programs. Family practice achieved remarkable success in a relatively short period of time. By 1978, 85% of all U.S. medical schools either had, or were in the process of developing, a department of division of family practice (Table 4.5). Residencies proliferated. While in 1969 there were 15 programs in family practice, by 1977 the number had increased to 325. The number of residents increased from 0 in 1968 to 5421 in 1977 (Table 4.6). After 1976 the number of residents in family practice exceeded those in pediatrics.

Family practice programs became more popular with medical students. A survey of students at the State University of New York Upstate Medical Center (Oates and Feldman, 1974) found a shift between 1967–1968 and 1972 in career interests from other specialties to family practice. The percentage of students expressing an interest in family practice rose

Table 4.5. Organizational Units for Family Practice in
            Medical Schools: 1978

Unit	Number
Departments	84
Divisions	13
Other programs	4
Departments under development	9
Schools without activity	21
Total	131

Source: Geyman (1978:595).

Table 4.6. Number of Family Practice Residency Programs and Residents

Year	Number of FP Residency Programs	Number of FP Residents	Number of Pediatric Residents
1969	15	0	
1970	45	290	2592
1971	62	532	2844
1972	117	1015	3238
1973	164	1771	4231
1974	205	2671	4784
1975	232	3720	4906
1976	278	4675	5028
1977	325	4966	4734
1978	343	6000	5331
1979	366	6352	5603
1980	380	6344	5171
1981	385	7004	5961
1982	388	7040	5720
1983	388	7236	6140
1984	386	7588	6091

Sources: Geyman (1978:595); *Journal of the AMA* (1982:3271; 1984:1546, 1548; 1985:1587, 1589; 1986:1586).

from 4% in a series of 1967–1968 surveys, to 17% in 1972. Family practice, along with internal medicine, was the only specialty that gained in popularity. Other specialties, including most notably pediatrics, declined during the same period (Table 4.7).

At Jefferson Medical College in Philadelphia, the percentage of students interested in family practice as a career increased from 6.3% in 1971 to 7.1% in 1972 and 7.4% in 1973. The figure almost doubled to

Table 4.7. SUNY Medical Student Career Choices in Two Surveys

Choice	1967–1968[a]	1972	Change
None	33	30	−3
Surgery	20	16	−4
Internal medicine	14	21	+7
Pediatrics	10	7	−3
Psychiatry	6	2	−4
Family practice	4	17	+13
Radiology	4	1	−3
Obstetrics/gynecology	3	1	−2
Other	6	4	−2
Total	100	100	

[a] This figure represents (in percentages) averages calculated for the 1967 and 1968 surveys.
Source: Oates and Feldman (1974:563).

14.7% in 1974 and rose again to 17.3% in 1975 (Herman and Veloski, 1977). No other specialty experienced an increase. Pediatrics declined from 9.2% in 1971 to 8.7% in 1975 (Table 4.8).

A study (Fishman and Zimet, 1972) of first-year medical students toward five medical specialties found that family practice ranked the highest at 25%, followed by surgery (23%), internal medicine (20%), pediatrics (19%), and psychiatry (13%).

Another indicator of the growing popularity of family practice was the demand for residency positions. In 1978, 94% of the 2183 first-year residency positions in family practice were filled. Given the logistical problems involved in matching applicants with positions, anything over 90% usually qualifies as complete (Willard and Ruhe, 1978). In fact, there were more students applying for the residency positions than the programs could accommodate. In the same year, medical schools reported that between 15 and 35% of their graduates were entering family practice (Geyman, 1978:596).

The caliber of student in family practice also improved. Through the 1950s and 1960s, students opting for general practice were not as capable as their colleagues. A 1964 study (Schumacher, 1964) compared the aptitude of interns in five groups, those intending to practice in the areas of (1) general medicine, (2) internal medicine, or (3) surgery, and those intending to combine part-time practice with academic careers in either (4) medicine or (5) surgery. The study measured aptitude in terms of students' performance on the verbal and scientific parts of the standardized Medical College Admissions Test (MCATs). The results showed that those with career plans in general medicine were at the bottom of both scales; those aspiring to academic careers were at the top; those

Table 4.8. Distribution of Residency Preferences of Students at Jefferson Medical College[a]

	Year of Graduation				
Residency Preference	1971	1972	1973	1974	1975
Family Medicine	6.3	7.1	7.4	14.7	17.3
Internal medicine	30.4	31.1	32.8	32.7	29.3
Pediatrics	9.2	8.8	6.2	6.2	8.7
Surgery	21.3	19.4	19.8	19.2	12.0
Obstetrics/gynecology	5.2	7.1	5.6	5.1	5.3
Psychiatry	6.9	0.6	8.6	6.8	2.4
Other	17.8	21.2	19.6	11.9	23.1
Undecided or none	2.9	4.7	0.0	3.4	1.9
Total	100	100	100	100	100

[a] In percentages.
Source: Herman and Veloski (1977:103).

wanting to pursue full-time specialty careers were in the middle. A decade later, another study (Herman and Veloski, 1977) found that the aptitude of students indicating a preference for family practice, as measured by the academic performance and their scores on the National Board Examinations, the examinations that medical students take at the end of their undergraduate medical training, was comparable to that of all other students, with the exception of those interested in internal medicine, who performed significantly better and those in psychiatry who performed significantly worse (Table 4.9).

Finally, once in practice, family practitioners, unlike their counterparts in pediatrics, were satisfied with both the training they had received as students and with their career choices. In a national survey of 876 residency-trained family practitioners (McCranie, Hornsby, and Cavert, 1982), 72% of practitioners claimed they were "very satisfied" with their training; another 22% were "moderately satisfied;" only 6% expressed dissatisfaction. Sixty percent indicated that they were "very satisfied" with their work in general; another 35% were "moderately satisfied;" only 5% were "dissatisfied."

FROM SHORTAGE TO SURPLUS

The flurry of activity through the 1960s and 1970s to increase the number of health care providers, including the rapid expansion in medical education, was so successful it resulted in a complete turnaround in

Table 4.9. Residency Preferences and Acadmeic Performance of Students at Jefferson Medical College

Residency Preference	Mean Grade-Point Average By School Year			Mean National Board Scores Part		
	First	Second	Third	I	II	III
Family practice	83.1	81.3	83.3	513	530	521
Internal medicine	84.8[a]	83.1[a]	84.7[a]	542[a]	560[a]	559[a]
Pediatrics	83.5	81.4	84.4[a]	519	541	513
Surgery	83.5	82.1	84.6	521	522	504
Obstetrics/gynecology	82.1	80.5	83.5	472[b]	495[b]	451[b]
Psychiatry	80.9[b]	79.4[b]	82.3[b]	467[b]	473[b]	428[b]
Other	83.8	82.4[a]	84.2[a]	519	537	500
Overall mean	83.7	82.1	84.2	522	536	516

[a] Significantly greater than family practice.
[b] Significantly less than family practice.
Source: Herman and Veloski (1977:103).

the physician supply problem. By the mid-1970s health care analysts were talking not about a shortage of doctors, but a surplus. In 1976, the Carnegie Commission on Policy—an influential advisory group—reversed the position it had taken in 1970 and began warning of a serious upcoming oversupply problem. In the same year, the Department of Health, Education and Welfare established the Graduate Medical Education National Advisory Committee (GMENAC) to systematically study the confusing health manpower situation. GMENAC predicted that on the basis of current trends, there would be an overall surplus of about 70,000 doctors by 1990. A small number of specialties, the Committee pointed out, including emergency medicine, preventive medicine, general psychiatry, and notably, child psychiatry, would experience a shortage. The rest, including pediatrics, were headed for a surplus.

GMENAC calculated a precise surplus of almost 5000 pediatricians (Table 4.10). But this figure actually masks the seriousness of the problem for general or primary care pediatrics because it calculates the net surplus for both general pediatrics and pediatric subspecialties combined. The breakdown according to areas of pediatrics indicated that while most pediatric subspecialties would not be able to meet their manpower requirements, general pediatrics would experience a surplus of close to 7500 practitioners (Table 4.11). Matched with projections for the number of children, estimates showed that the ratio of pediatricians to children would more than double between 1975 and 1990, from 1:3273 to 1:1356 (Table 4.12; the ratios are plotted in Figure 4.1).

Though pediatricians challenged GMENAC's numbers, they were taken aback by the implications of the report and could scarcely believe their predicament. "It seems like just yesterday," wrote one incredulous pediatrician, Abraham Bergman (1974:533), "[that there were] dire pronouncements about the child-health manpower shortage. The 'pediatric numbers game' was worked to prove that since fewer kids' doctors were going to be around to see more kids, pediatricians couldn't possibly carry the whole load." Bergman admitted that he had been among those who, earlier in the decade, had called on other groups, including PNPs, to become involved in the child health care. "Well, it worked," he continued, "the crisis cries were heeded. . . . Such profound changes have taken place in the manpower game, that general pediatricians in the United States may well be teetering on the threshold of a museum" (Bergman, 1974:533).

PNPS AS A THREAT

Besides the problem of numbers, pediatricians were disturbed by the growing independence of PNPs. Until the mid-1970s the movement had

Table 4.10. Projected Requirements and Supply for Selected Specialties

Specialty	Supply	Requirements	Surplus (Shortage)
All doctors	535,750	466,000	69,750
General psychiatry	30,500	38,500	(8,000)
Child psychiatry	4,100	9,000	(4,900)
Emergency medicine	9,250	13,500	(4,250)
Preventive medicine	5,550	7,300	(1,750)
Anesthesiology	19,450	21,000	(1,550)
Physical medicine and rehab.	2,400	3,200	(800)
Haematology/oncology	8,300	9,000	(700)
Dermatology	7,350	6,950	400
Gastroenterology	6,900	6,500	400
Otolaryngology	8,500	8,000	500
Thoracic surgery	2,900	2,050	850
Infectious diseases	3,250	2,250	1,000
Allergy-immunology	3,050	2,050	1,000
Osteopathic general practice	23,850	22,000	1,150
Plastic surgery	3,900	2,700	1,200
Rheumatology	3,000	1,700	1,300
Urology	9,350	7,700	1,650
Endocrinology	3,850	2,050	1,800
Nephrology	4,850	2,750	2,100
Neurosurgery	8,650	2,650	2,450
Family practice	64,400	61,300	3,100
Neurology	8,650	5,500	3,150
Pulmonary diseases	6,950	3,600	3,350
Pathology	16,850	13,500	3,350
General internal medicine	73,800	70,250	3,550
Ophthalmology	16,300	11,600	4,700
General pediatrics and sub-specialties	41,350	36,400	4,950
Orthopedic surgery	20,100	15,100	5,000
Cardiology	14,900	7,750	7,150
Radiology	27,800	18,000	9,800
Obstetrics/gynecology	34,450	24,000	10,450
General surgery	35,300	23,500	11,800

Source: Adapted from AAP (1981a:589)

focused principally on working with the medical profession to legitimize the nurse practitioner role and to prove that nurse practitioners could deliver quality health care. As the movement gained strength and confidence, however, PNPs, along with other nurse practitioners, prepared to take the next step in their professional development. They sought to consolidate their position in the health care system. Their central focus shifted from recognition to greater status, income, and security (Ford, 1982; Lewis, 1982).

Table 4.11. Projected Requirements and Supply for Pediatrics

	Supply	Requirements	Surplus (Shortage)
General pediatrics	37,750	30,250	7,500
Pediatric allergy	900	900	—
Pediatric cardiology	1,000	1,150	(150)
Pediatric endocrinology	250	800	(550)
Pediatric hematology/oncology	550	1,650	(1,100)
Pediatric nephrology	200	350	(150)
Neonatology	700	1,300	(600)
Total pediatrics	41,350	36,400	4,950

Source: Adapted from AAP (1981a:589).

Nurse practitioners began to assume greater control over their own training and used that control to upgrade their education. The first nurse practitioner programs were clinically oriented, certificate-granting, continuing education courses offered in a variety of settings including hospitals, schools of medicine, and schools of nursing, and codirected by nurses and doctors. By the mid-1970s there was a discernible trend toward programs in schools of nursing run by nurses alone and leading to a Master of Science in Nursing (Kahn, 1979). In the area of pediatrics alone, for example, the number of certificate PNP programs decreased from 42 in 1973 to 22 in 1980, while the number of Master's programs increased from eight in 1973 to 21 in 1980 (Butler, 1984:187–188). By 1982 most of these Master's programs (58%) were directed exclusively by a PNP, while only 42% were codirected by a PNP and a pediatrician (Bullough et al., 1984:193).

Table 4.12. Number of Pediatricians, Number of Children,[a] and Ratio

Year	Pediatricians	Children	Ratio
1960	—	69.0	—
1965	—	76.7	—
1970	18,819	77.1	4,096
1975	22,730	74.4	3,273
1980	29,462	72.5	2,460
1985	35,617	70.3	1,973
1990[b]	52,780	71.6	1,356
2000[b]	59,659	74.8	1.254

[a] In millions.
[b] Projected.
Sources: AMA Council on Long Range Planning and Development (1987:242); Budetti (1981:599, 601); Gorwitz and Smith (1975:592).

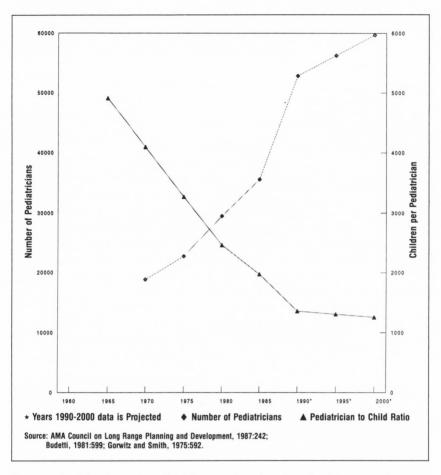

Figure 4.1. Number of pediatricians and ratio of pediatricians to children. *Sources*: AMA Council on Long Range Planning and Development (1987:242); Budetti (1981:599); Gorwitz and Smith (1975).

Nurse practitioners also created their own professional organizations. In 1974 PNPs formed the National Association of Pediatric Nurse Associates and Practitioners (NAPNAP) and the Association of Faculties of PNP/A Programs (AFPNP/AP). There were similar groups for nurse practitioners in other areas of practice. Working together with the ANA, these groups introduced a standardized certification system for nurse practitioners, much like the specialty boards in medicine. They lobbied for legal changes to accommodate their expanded scope of practice. Between 1971 and 1985, 38 states changed their laws to authorize nurses to diagnose and treat disease (Moloney, 1986:189). Five states (Alaska, Idaho, New Mexico, Oregon, and Washington) gave nurse practitioners full authority to prescribe medications. Another eight states (North Carolina, Kentucky, Maine, New Hampshire, New York, Mississippi, Utah, and California) granted nurse practitioners partial prescribing authority. In Mississippi, PNPs won the legal right to prescribe drugs, while other nurse practitioners could not (Weston, 1984:6). But the ultimate legal goal of nurse practitioners was, and still is, the right to practice independently without the supervision of doctors.

As they watched these developments, pediatricians could see a confrontation coming: "A struggle for patients and dollars," wrote Bergman (1974:534) in his analysis of the oversupply problem, "couched, of course, in more respectable terms appears inevitable." The cooperation that once characterized the relationship between PNPs and pediatricians disappeared. In 1975 the AAP, which had once so enthusiastically supported PNPs, decided to "clarify" its position with respect to the PNPs proper scope or practice. It issued a policy statement in which it expressly opposed the idea of PNPs in free-standing, independent practices:

> The scope of practice of the PNA/P is based on a common understanding by physicians and nurses providing child health care that an appropriately educated nurse can competently deliver certain medical services traditionally performed by the physician. But provision of these services is still the responsibility of the physician and must be performed under his direction and supervision, and review. (AAP, 1975)

Pediatricians insisted that PNPs had neither the training nor the expertise to function independently, despite the fact that their own studies, produced to promote the PNP concept when it was first introduced, showed that PNPs could, in fact, effectively manage much of the day-to-day work of primary care pediatrics.

The AAP also created an Ad Hoc Committee to reexamine its position on nurse practitioners and other types of "physician extenders." Sensitive to the potential danger that such groups posed and concerned about the effects of an increasingly crowded pediatric turf, the AAP, acting on the Committee's recommendations, issued another policy statement stipulating that pediatricians were categorically opposed to the development of any additional category of pediatric personnel (Van Gelder, 1978:8).

Another sign of the growing tensions between pediatricians and PNPs was the rift that developed between the AAP and the ANA. In 1969 the two organizations had established a liaison committee to develop the standardized certification system for PNPs. The pediatric representatives on the committee, in 1973, agreed to an arrangement whereby the system would be administered entirely by the nurses themselves and pediatricians would participate only in the testing of candidates. In spite of the agreement, the AAP unilaterally pulled out of the plan, insisting that its representative be allowed on the certification board itself and on any committee working at the policy-making level. Robert Frazier, the AAP's Executive Director, argued that without such representation the AAP could not recommend PNPs to its membership or the families they served. The ANA described the move as "an attempt by one profession to control another" and moved ahead with its plans to implement the certification system (*American Journal of Nursing*, 1974:388).

But the most powerful tool that pediatricians had against PNPs was the fact that large numbers of PNPs still depended on them for employment. After 1975 pediatricians slowed their hiring. NAPNAP surveys show that fewer PNPs were employed 6 months after graduation in 1982 (67%) than had been the case in 1974 (73%); more 1982 graduates were employed in non-PNP roles (18%) than 1974 graduates (14%); and salary gains for PNPs, though in line with the Consumer Price Index over the years 1974–1982, had not been as great as for other nurse practitioners. All of these factors made the profession less appealing. Predictably, the number of PNP programs and the total number of students in these programs also declined after 1975, both in absolute terms and as a percentage of the total number of nurse practitioner programs and students. In 1973 there were 50 PNP programs in the country and they accounted for 38% of all nurse practitioner programs. By 1980, there were only 43 PNP programs, accounting for 22% of all programs. In 1973 there were 381 registered PNP students, accounting for 35% of all nurse practitioner students. By 1980, there were only 290, accounting for 18% of all students (Bullough et al., 1984:194). Though they did not thwart the PNP movement completely, pediatricians were able to slow it down somewhat.

FAMILY PRACTICE AS A THREAT

The advantage that pediatricians had over PNPs was that, as doctors, they could assert their professional dominance (Freidson, 1970b) over the less powerful nurses. In family practitioners, who were equal members of the medical profession, pediatricians had a more formidable challenge. The goals of the first family practitioners, as they concerned the child health market, were relatively modest. They wanted a place, alongside pediatricians and other health care workers, in the primary care of children. But by the mid-1970s some family practitioners wanted to see their specialty displace pediatrics altogether. Cooptation, not cooperation, was the goal toward which they felt family practice should be striving. Edmund Pellegrino (1978), for example, a leading family practitioner, argued that family practitioners were better doctors for children because they were trained to take the child's family relationships and environmental influences into account and could therefore provide more complete and comprehensive care. If pediatricians wanted to continue to provide primary care for children, he suggested, they would have to abandon the pediatric model that treated the child as an individual patient, and augment their knowledge and skills in family care. In other words, they would have to become family practitioners. In considering the relationship between family practice and not only pediatrics, but internal medicine, where a similar turf battle was playing itself out in relation to adult health care, Pellegrino (1978:134) predicted: "It is more likely that general internal medicine and pediatrics will merge gradually with family medicine, and that much of the current stress among them will be slowly dissipated."

Pediatrics did not initially oppose the organization of the family practice movement, possibly because they did not anticipate its rapid growth and popularity, or perhaps because in the context of manpower shortages, they felt there were too few pediatricians to meet the growing demand for pediatric services. As Bergman (1974) noted, in the late 1960s pediatricians were eager for other groups to help them pull the primary care load. But with an imminent oversupply problem and family practitioners more aggressively pursuing the child health care market, pediatricians began to perceive family practitioners as competitors, and the competition between pediatrics and family practice as a zero-sum game. To the extent that family practitioners succeeded in making gains as child health care providers, pediatricians lost. Pediatrics began to take a firm and unequivocal stand against *any* involvement of family practitioners in child health care. In 1975, John MacQueen (1975:25), president of the AAP and a pediatrician who had been one of the first educators involved in training family practice residents in pediatric techniques, stated that pediatrics would not "support or participate in a restructuring or artificial stratification of American medicine to conform to the stated expectations of the generally trained physician." Pediatricians, he argued, because of their training, interest, and experience in the care of children both in health and illness, were better equipped than family practitioners to provide child health care services and should be managing most, if not all, child health care. He proposed as a goal for the AAP that "within the next twenty years, the great majority of all children in this nation shall have access to the quality care provided by pediatricians" (MacQueen, 1975:25). Others (Olmsted, 1979:11; Van Gelder, 1978:8) resurrected the "children are not miniature adults" argument that the founders of pediatrics had used to rationalize the creation of pediatrics as a distinct branch of medicine. Family practitioners could simply not compete with the years of specialized training and experience that pediatricians brought to their practices. In 1981, the AAP set up a Task Force on the Promotion of Pediatrics to convince the public that pediatricians, and not family practitioners, were "the best qualified providers of care for children and adolescents" (Blim, 1981:2). In 1982, the AAP retained the services of Daniel J. Edelman, Inc., a leading public relations firm, to assist in this promotional initiative.

WHO DOES IT BETTER?: A DEBATE BETWEEN PEDIATRICS AND FAMILY PRACTICE

As Pellegrino (1978) and MacQueen's (1975) remarks demonstrate, the territorial dispute between pediatrics and family practice was cast in terms of which specialty was best able to provide primary care to children. In 1984 the Department of Pediatrics at the University of Rochester Strong Memorial Hospital Medical Center sponsored a debate on the question: "Who should provide primary health care to children: pediatricians or family medicine physicians?" The debate captures the central arguments and rhetoric that each specialty used to assert its exclusive claims over child health care. The debate demonstrates that both specialties argued that their interest in children was comprehensive, that is, that they could satisfy the full range of child health care needs, both those that were medical and those that affected their psychosocial functioning. From the point of view of pediatrics, it was the "new pediatrics," as it was ostensibly being practiced by pediatricians, that made pediatricians the better health care providers for children. The dispute with family practice then, gave pediatricians an even greater stake in the new pediatrics.

James E. Strain spoke on behalf of pediatricians. In 1984, at the time of the debate, Strain was a clinical professor of pediatrics at the University of Colorado and was serving as president of the AAP. Michael Klein, a pediatrician-turned-family practitioner, spoke for family practice. The circumstances of Klein's conversion to family practice are worth noting, because they so clearly illustrate the pediatrician's fundamental dilemma. Klein received his medical degree from Stanford University in 1966 and was his class's recipient of the pediatric Harold K. Kaiser Award.

After his internship at Bronx Municipal Hospital Center at Albert Einstein University, he completed a pediatric residency at the Montreal Children's Hospital. In 1970 he took a position as Fellow in Ambulatory Pediatrics at the University of Rochester and between 1971 and 1975 served as the medical director of a community health clinic in Rochester. As director, he employed several family practitioners. He felt that a multispecialty practice model, with family practitioners and a nurse practitioner serving on the front line while pediatricians, obstetricians, internists, and community mental health workers handled referrals, would maximize the efficiency of the clinic. Along with administrative duties, Klein expected to provide part-time pediatric consultation for the family practitioners on staff, and also to do some well-child care.

Klein soon discovered that the family practitioners rarely needed his assistance. Of the few consultations that did come his way, Klein observed:

> But I had the feeling that [they] were really designed to make me feel good, because I was there and they didn't want me to be unhappy. If I hadn't been there, they could have gone to Strong Memorial Hospital and gotten a proper pediatric subspecialty consult without any problem. They needed pediatric subspecialists, not pediatric generalists. (Hoekelman, Klein, and Strain, 1984:468)

Klein felt no more useful in the area of well-child care. At first he alternated well-child visits with the clinic nurse practitioner. But she was increasingly able to manage on her own. The family practitioners provided whatever backup she needed for diagnostic and serious problems. Feeling squeezed out of any significant role in providing health care, Klein reassessed his career goals:

> At that point, I had several options. I could quit; I could administrate full time; or I could dig in and become a proper family doctor. I chose the latter, and over the next four years, I had a personal tutorial from the family doctors whom I'd hired. I did the rare consultation for them, but the tables were decidedly turned. (Hoekelman et al., 1984:468)

Klein formalized the switch by seeking certification from both the recently formed American Board of Family Practice and the College of Family Physicians of Canada. At the time of the debate he was the Director of the Department of Family Medicine at the Sir Mortimer B. Davis Jewish General Hospital in Montreal, and a professor of both family medicine and pediatrics at the McGill University School of Medicine.

The Case for Pediatrics

In presenting the case for pediatrics, Strain adopted a rhetoric strongly reminiscent of the arguments that an earlier generation of pediatricians had used in trying to establish pediatrics as a distinct specialty— that a *generalist* was no match for the specialty trained and oriented pediatrician. There were fundamental differences, Strain contended, between generalists like family practitioners and pediatricians, "differences in training, experiences, interest and outlook . . . differences [that] make pediatricians better qualified to provide comprehensive care for the children in our society" (Hoekelman et al., 1984:463).

Strain focused first on the training that each specialty provided for its residents, contrasting the 3 years of specialized training that pediatricians received—all of it concentrated on children—with the 6 months or less that most family practice programs devoted to the pediatric component of their students' training. He emphasized, in particular, the comprehensiveness of pediatricians' training. He pointed to growth and development, preventive medicine, anticipatory guidance, the care of the handicapped and chronically ill child, and psychosocial disorders as "the most significant unmet health care needs in the child and adolescent populations" (Hoekelman et al., 1984:463). Training in such areas, he maintained, took time—time that the resident in family practice simply did not have. Though most pediatric programs were themselves still ambivalent about the "new pediatrics" and had in fact introduced only minimal changes in their curricula in the direction of a more comprehensive pediatrics, Strain insisted that pediatricians were being trained more completely in these areas than were family practitioners.

The "information gap" between pediatricians and family practitioners that started in residency training, Strain continued, extended into practice. He cited data showing that pediatricians spent 98% of their time treating individuals who were 21 years of age and under, while family practitioners spent only 24% of their time with this age group and the remainder of their time treating adults. The constant and exclusive exposure of pediatricians to children and their problems, he reasoned, gave them a clear edge over the family practitioner. It produced a "sixth sense" about children that family practitioners lacked, a sense that allowed them to spot problems before they escalated into more serious difficulties.

In their continuing education, family practitioners had to keep up with the literature on the health problems of all age groups while pediatricians were free to focus on children and adolescents alone. To illustrate his point, Strain contrasted the number of articles about a range of childhood health risks in the official publications of each specialty. Between 1980 and 1982, the AAP's publication *Pediatrics* carried 43 articles on childhood accidents and accident prevention while the *Journal of Family Practice* carried only five. *Pediatrics* published 24 articles on sudden infant death syndrome while the *Journal of Family Practice* carried none. There had been 17 articles on care of the handicapped child in *Pediatrics* and only five in the *Journal of Family Practice.* "This is not an indictment of the continuing education efforts of family practice," Strain clarified (Hoekelman et al., 1984:464). The continuing education programs of family practice were not designed to cover pediatric care as completely or as comprehensively as the programs for pediatricians.

Addressing head-on perhaps the strongest suit held by family practitioners, Strain commented on the special relationship that pediatricians had, not only with their young patients, but with their families. Pediatricians were taught, he asserted, that children were products of their environments and understood the importance of dealing with their health needs in the context of their families and communities. Though their therapeutic focus might be the child, pediatricians did have an appreciation for, and an ability to deal with, the broader forces that influence children's lives so profoundly. In their counseling work and in treating psychosocial disorders pediatricians did adopt a family- and community-oriented approach.

Finally, Strain discussed the differences between the two specialties in terms of their interest in the problems of children. He elaborated on pediatrics' long tradition of advocacy on children's behalf in a broad range of areas including child abuse and neglect, automobile-restraint laws and accident prevention more generally, health care funding and facilities, and education of the handicapped child. Children could not vote, he pointed out, and many could not even speak on their own behalf. Pediatricians, because of their special relationship with children, had always been willing to fill that role and had a unique commitment to child advocacy. He concluded:

> I have spoken of the pediatrician's advantage in training and experience when it comes to child health care, but there is no way to quantify the level of interest and dedication that comes from choosing to spend your professional life helping children. It is a feeling that all pediatricians have. It is the reason we become pediatricians in the first place, and it is the reason why I believe pediatricians should continue to provide comprehensive, primary health care to our children. (Hoekelman et al., 1984:467)

Strain advised family practitioners to look elsewhere for patients. With the rapid aging of the population, there would be a tremendous need for health care services among the elderly, he observed. Family practitioners, with the bulk of their training and experience in the care of adults, were the "logical" providers of these services. For infants, children, and young adults, pediatricians were clearly the optimum health care providers and should be the physicians of choice.

The Case for Family Practice

Klein presented a more restrained and moderate position for family practice than Pellegrino or other family practitioners might have, probably because despite his conversion to family practice he was still, in a sense, among colleagues and friends at the Rochester debate. He did make the point that by treating the family as its therapeutic unit, family practice had a distinct advantage over pediatricians in caring for children. Good pediatricians, he conceded, had always attempted to take the family into consideration in their dealings with children. "But it is a struggle for them," he argued, "and the context has to be created. Family physicians, on the other hand, have the context already built into their basic practices" (Hoekelman et al., 1984:468). He suggested, as well, that because primary care pediatricians depended so heavily on well-child visits to support their practices, they might be encouraging more such visits than were actually necessary, and, in the process, undermining the development of parental confidence and competence.

But for the most part, rather than argue that family practitioners were better than pediatricians at meeting child health care needs, Klein took issue only with the notion that pediatricians, and pediatricians alone, should provide child health care services. "I freely admit," he started by saying (Hoekelman et al., 1984:467), "that most office-based pediatricians know how to care for children, but it does not follow that family physicians do not, and in fact, the whole debate makes me extremely uncomfortable."

Klein singled out the AAP for attempting to block the development of family practice and for escalating an unhealthy competition between the two specialties. Though the AAP maintained that it was opposing family practice in the interests of children, the conflict between pediatrics and family practice, Klein insisted, was not about the quality of care provided to children, but one of politics and economics—"dividing up the shrinking pie." The AAP, he observed, was concerned about the future of general pediatrics. Pediatricians were threatened in the area of primary care by PNPs and family practitioners, and in the area of treating sick children by pediatric subspecialties. But in response to those threats, he charged, the organization was guilty of putting pediatricians' interests before the good of the children they professed to serve. "Dr. Strain has told you," he said (Hoekelman et al., 1984:467), "that all children need or deserve a pediatrician. Perhaps what he really means is that all pediatricians need or deserve enough child patients to make a living." The policies of the AAP, he asserted, were aimed to keep child health care the exclusive preserve of pediatricians, despite the evidence that other groups could function at least as effectively in this area. He accused the AAP of abandoning its long and noble tradition of child advocacy. Referring to the AAP's campaign against family practice, he declared (Hoekelman et al., 1984:469): "This is not child advocacy; this is pediatrician advocacy, and I don't think the Academy ought to feel very good about that."

Klein questioned whether the AAP's goal of a pediatrician for every child was realistic, given the numbers of pediatricians that would be required and the child population needed to support a pediatric practice, especially in rural areas. Most smaller communities, he argued, could not sustain a primary care pediatrician. He questioned how committed pediatricians were to providing the comprehensive care that Strain described. He pointed out, quite accurately, that neither pediatric educators nor most pediatricians in private, primary care practices were demonstrating much interest in the nonmedical problems of children and adolescents.

Klein concluded by suggesting that pediatricians reassess their priorities and that they put the needs of children before those of the profession:

> I believe that unless we move in positive ways and do more than deal with the issue by means of public relations, there will be a level of interspecialty conflict that will diminish the effectiveness of all physicians and lead to increased cost to society. We are all too aware that physicians naturally expand services to maximize or maintain an acceptable income. The challenge is to resist this and look to the needs of society. (Hoekelman et al., 1984:475)

He proposed that rather than looking at child health care from the perspective of their respective specialties, both pediatrics and family practice adopt a community perspective—one in which all primary care physicians would work together, forming logical bridges between their specialties, in an effort to provide community-oriented, rather than profession-oriented care to children.

PEDIATRIC OPTIONS

As pediatricians confronted increased competition, the inevitable questions about the specialty's future resurfaced. "Pediatrics is on the verge of an identity crisis" declared one pediatrician (Kotch, 1976:9). "Do we really need more pediatricians?" asked another rhetorically (Haggerty, 1972:682). Certainly not, he responded, if pediatricians continued to do what they had done in the past. On the other hand, he added, if they were willing to change—to "take on some of the new roles society is asking of them" and to meet "those needs of children never yet adequately met—the consequences of developmental, behavioral and social problems" (1972:683), there would be opportunities for growth. Haggerty (1974) advised the specialty to take a proactive, rather than reactive, stance:

> While we are not masters of our own fate, we can be and should be a part of this process of determining what our job in the community is going to be. Together with the consumer, and with the other health professions, we will not only improve health more in the future, but we will have a better time doing it if we move into some of these new roles. (Haggerty, 1974:549)

Ivan Pless, an associate professor of pediatrics, prevention, and community health at the University of Rochester, after a thorough analysis of the trends likely to influence the future course of the specialty, came to the same conclusion. "From the viewpoint of the epidemiologist's ivory tower," he wrote (1974:223), "the future of pediatrics looks bleak." The falling birth rate, the decline in infectious diseases, the referral of many difficult but interesting cases to subspecialists, the consequences of increasing pediatric manpower, and finally the growth of family medicine and allied health personnel all made an examination of primary care pediatrics, in Pless' words, "a matter of urgency."

According to Pless, there were three directions that pediatrics could follow: increased, shifting, or decreased professionalization. Drawing on the sociological work on professions, especially Eliot Freidson's contributions (1970a), Pless defined "professionalization" as the amount of technical expertise connected to the work of an occupation. Increased professionalization involved the evolution of pediatricians into consultants,. working on a referral basis, on problems that required highly specialized skills and technical competence. This would mean leaving primary care to family and general practitioners, and various types of allied health personnel. Although a consulting model did not necessarily imply subspecialization, Pless felt that for most young pediatricians this would be advisable. He also observed that this option would require little restructuring in medical training, since control over pediatric education was in the hands of pediatric subspecialties anyway.

Shifting professionalization referred to greater involvement in treating the family, rather than simply children. Pless urged pediatricians to give serious consideration to this option because of the possibility that "it may be forced upon us as a matter of necessity" (Pless, 1974:236). He conceded that there were advantages to the family practice model with its emphasis on the interaction between health and illness, and the family, the community, and the environment. But he also raised the question of whether the model of practice it implied needed to be the new discipline of family practice or whether it could be viewed as a modification or subspecialty of pediatrics.

Decreasing professionalization meant that pediatricians would expand their activities to meet what Pless called "the full spectrum of children's health needs" (Pless, 1974:237). He identified several areas of expansion: learning and behavioral problems, school health, accident prevention, child abuse, sudden infant death syndrome, drug, sex, and family counseling, and the management of the psychological and social consequences of chronic illness.

Pless referred to this option as "decreasing" professionalization because it would involve pediatricians in activities that did not fit the familiar mold of medical care. There was the possibility, therefore, of reduced professional status, certainly in the eyes of their more "hard-nosed, subspecialty colleagues" and possibly even among the public, who might not accept pediatricians in this role. Pediatricians would have to ensure that their performance in these areas was not "amateurish." To be responsible for something, Pless insisted, "involves a knowledge of the area and some basic skill in it" (Pless, 1974:238). Pediatricians would need to retool:

> *Much* more emphasis must be given to communication skill; to an understanding of the interaction of psychosocial, genetic, and environmental factors with the disease process; to the organization, politics and economics of medical care delivery; to the sociology and psychology of the family unit; to child development and behavior; to the community and its resources; and above all, to the potential roles of paraprofessionals, nonprofessionals, and laymen themselves. (Pless, 1974:238)

Pless went on to describe how pediatricians might include social workers among their office staff to deal with children's social problems—or in cases where families would have difficulty bearing the additional cost of a social worker—how lay persons, chiefly middle-class mothers, might be recruited for the task. Lay "family counselors," as he called them, "represent an important new manpower resource to assist the pediatrician in expanding his role in this area" (Pless, 1974:241).

Of the three alternatives he outlined, decreasing professionalization, in Pless' view, demanded the most radical restructuring of pediatric training programs. But it was also the only option that offered any hope of preserving pediatrics as a distinct, primary care specialty. This may explain why, despite its attendant risks, organized pediatrics seems to have staked its future on an expansion into new areas of care.

Chapter 5

Redefining Pediatrics

INTRODUCTION

The movement toward the new pediatrics that started with the dissatisfied pediatrician syndrome was invigorated through the supply crisis of the 1970s. More convinced than ever that the survival of pediatrics as a primary care specialty depended on a reorientation toward a more comprehensive model of practice, many of the specialty's leaders continued to support the new pediatrics.

So too did those who were developing careers studying and teaching the new pediatrics. This group included both academic generalists and the graduates of the few fellowship programs in behavioral and adolescent medicine that pediatric departments had instituted through the 1960s. Gradually these "new pediatricians" created organizations through which they promoted the integration of the behavioral problems of children and adolescents into general pediatrics. One of these organizations was the Ambulatory Pediatric Association (APA). In the late 1950s, academic generalists began meeting informally at APS and SPR meetings. In 1960 these academics joined with pediatricians working in neighborhood health centers, in health departments, and in private practice to create the APA. Though the organization eventually opened its membership to nurses, social workers, psychologists, and sociologists concerned with child health care issues, pediatricians still make up the vast majority of its membership (Alpert, 1995). Over the next 15 years more specialized groups also formed, including the Society for Adolescent Medicine in 1968, the Society for Developmental Pediatrics in 1978, and the Society for Behavioral Pediatrics in 1983.

Besides these groups, the AAP was a central player in the promotion of the new pediatrics. After 1960, the AAP created scores of organizational subgroups—councils, sections, committees—in areas such as community pediatrics, the psychosocial aspects of child and family health, mental growth and development, adoption and dependent care, children with handicaps, accident prevention, and environmental hazards. These subgroups examined child-related issues and made policy recommendations to the Executive Board of the AAP. They also prepared and distributed informational and educational materials for pediatricians, and ran courses and workshops.

While the crises and pressures described in previous chapters seemed to make the transformation of pediatrics imperative, this was no easy task. The new pediatrics proved difficult to translate into practice. Many among the research and teaching elite of the specialty were personally unaffected by the economic and existential crises of primary care pediatricians and remained committed to organically based education. And there were signs that primary care pediatricians themselves were not taking advantage of the opportunities that the new pediatrics provided. This chapter looks at these trends in practice and at the efforts of those who shared the vision of a more comprehensive pediatrics to steer the specialty more firmly in that direction.

LAGS IN PEDIATRIC PRACTICE

While at a programmatic level pediatrics became a specialty concerned with the behavioral and psychosocial aspects of children's development and adolescent health, practice patterns were slow to reflect the shift. Well into the 1980s figures showed that problems of a behavioral, psychosocial, or developmental nature did not comprise a significant proportion of pediatric practice. Such problems arose in between 5 to 40% of all visits to pediatricians. But behavioral problems were not among the top 10 or 20 diagnoses obtained in surveys of national samples of office-based pediatricians. The prevalence of diagnoses was only about 1.5%, even when second and third listed diagnoses were included (Starfield, 1982:379). As some of the "new pediatricians" saw it, although a mastery of developmental pediatrics was "an idea whose time has arrived . . . , its arrival has been not quite as soon as some would have liked and not without considerable resistance" (Richmond and Janis, 1983:15).

As part of their effort to promote the new pediatrics, groups such as the AAP targeted the public, hoping to create a more substantial market for pediatric services in these areas. In 1983, the AAP launched a public relations campaign designed to "dispel the image of the pediatrician as only a "baby doctor" and to educate the public about the services that can be provided by the pediatrician in the primary health care setting (Strain, 1983:442). The campaign emphasized the pediatrician's interest and expertise in dealing with problems of adolescence, care of the handicapped child, and sports medicine.

But it became increasingly obvious that the main impediment to a fuller integration of the new pediatrics had more to do with the reluctance of many primary care pediatricians to take on nonphysical problems rather than public perceptions about what pediatricians could do. Parents clearly wanted information about psychosocial issues (Hickson, Althemeir, and O'Connor, 1983) and the vast majority of them—in one study 82% (Deisher et al., 1965)—preferred to get that information from pediatricians. Indeed, most of the questions they wanted to direct to pediatricians dealt with psychosocial and behavioral issues, school problems, and the concerns of adolescents (Coleman, Patrick, and Baker, 1977; Goldberg et al., 1979; McCune, Richardson, and Powell, 1984; Starfield et al., 1980; Toister and Worley, 1976). The authors of one study concluded that "pediatric practice is a logical means of providing information to parents about their children's health, both behavioral and physical" (McCune et al., 1984:189).

Yet pediatricians consistently failed to respond to parental concerns about behavioral and psychosocial issues. Starfield and Borkowf (1969) found that pediatricians were much more likely to register awareness of a physical problem than a behavioral one. They recognized 90 out of 115 (78%) physical complaints, but only 20 out of 48 (42%) behavioral complaints. Behavioral complaints included "nervousness," an inability to get along with others, retardation, and school discipline problems. The severity of the behavioral problem did not explain the doctors' failure to respond, since some serious problems, such as fire-setting, were overlooked. Korsch et al. (1971) evaluated 450 well-child visits in both private and clinic settings, found that the behavioral aspects of pediatrics received only rudimentary and inferior responses from pediatricians, and that parents often left with their questions unanswered. In another study of 146 children with enuresis (a bed-wetting problem), teachers were better at recognizing the existence of problems that parents had mentioned in a medical history form, even though the pediatricians had access to the history forms completed by mothers and the teachers did not (Starfield and Sharp, 1971).

The implications for pediatrics were spelled out bluntly by Barbara Starfield, a long-time observer of patterns in pediatric practice: The specialty claimed to address not just childhood illnesses, but the full range of difficulties experienced by children and adolescents. It was using that claim to insist that pediatrics should continue to exist as a primary care specialty. It was lobbying federal and state governments for reimbursement policies more favorable to the provision of comprehensive and psychosocial care. But if pediatricians were counting on an image of themselves as comprehensive care-givers to save their specialty at the primary care level, they would need to do more than merely pay lip-

service to that image. They would need to start dealing with behavioral
and developmental problems.

> How can pediatricians justify their assertions that psychosocial problems
> and developmental concerns are a proper concern of pediatrics and worth
> reimbursement? . . . In this country pediatrics is, by custom, a primary
> care specialty. Continued claim to the characterization may require some
> hard thinking about the current status of the profession and its future.
> Appropriate solutions to these concerns can be addressed effectively only
> by a combined and concerted involvement of practitioners and academi-
> cians. The survival of the profession as a primary care discipline demands
> such attention. (Starfield, 1983:439)

One reason pediatricians failed to respond to behavioral complaints
was the extensive time and effort needed to treat such problems. Primary care pediatricians felt they needed to see as many patients as possible
and many had neither the time nor the inclination to become involved in
complicated behavioral complaints. Moreover, they were used to getting
quick results. "I was attracted into [pediatrics]," admitted one pediatrician (Haggerty, 1974:547), "because it was the kind of field where patients got well quickly, where I did not have to worry about 80-year-old
people who never seemed to get well. I suspect many pediatricians are
like this."

More fundamentally, analysts suggested, many practitioners did not
see psychosocial and behavioral problems as falling within the purview
of their medical practices and did not trust their skills when it came to
handling such problems (Haggerty, 1982; Starfield and Borkowf, 1969;
Thompson, 1984). These were the deeper attitudinal barriers that
needed to be overcome if the new pediatrics was ever to become a
reality.

The effort to redefine pediatrics involved three strategies. First, those
who believed in the new pediatrics sought to develop a more convincing
rationale to persuade practitioners that they had a role to play in taking
on children's nonphysical problems. Second, the reformers established
the new pediatrics more clearly and indisputably as the standard or
model of good pediatric practice. Finally, and most importantly, pediatric training programs had to be reformed. If primary care pediatricians
had trouble with the idea of treating psychosocial and behavioral problems, it was in large part because they were never trained for it. Pediatric
curricula continued to be organically oriented and the "thrills" for both
teachers and students were still in difficult diagnoses of physical illness and in quick, successful treatment. Pediatric education had to be
brought more clearly into line with what the advocates of the new pediatrics felt the practice of pediatrics ought to be. Practitioners needed to

be taught that their responsibilities extended beyond the physical problems of their patients and they needed to be given the skills to cope with the new demands being made of them.

A RATIONALE FOR THE NEW PEDIATRICS

The formulation of a rhetoric that defined and justified new roles for pediatricians started, as Chapter 3 shows, with the specialty's first foray into nontraditional aspects of care. The more committed the supporters of a new pediatrics became to a broader definition of their specialty, the more sophisticated the rhetoric. Proponents of the new pediatrics used a rhetoric of endangerment (Ibarra and Kitsuse, 1993:35)—they argued that negative childhood experiences were a serious threat, both over the short- and long-term, to children's well-being. They also used a rhetoric of entitlement (Ibarra and Kitsuse, 1993:34), insisting that all children had a right to a life free from the difficulties that might compromise their optimal growth and development.

Rates of venereal disease, mental illness, divorce, school absenteeism, drug abuse, and teenage pregnancies were all marshalled in support of the contention that there were vast numbers of troubled individuals in society. Many of their troubles, it was suggested, had their origins in the apparently trivial and often overlooked difficulties of childhood and adolescence. And even those behavioral problems that did not necessarily portend problems later in life caused discomfort in childhood and a disruption of family life, and school activities (Starfield, 1982). "The needs are vast," wrote one pediatrician (Cohen, 1984:791), "and often seriously unmet, and the resultant disabilities on the lives and potential of our children are very significant."

But the real issue that the promoters of the new pediatrics needed to address was the specialty's responsibility for the psychosocial difficulties of children. After all, no one disputed that children had needs in these areas or even that neglecting these needs had serious consequences. What some pediatricians did dispute was the suggestion that pediatrics had a role to play in the resolution of these problems.

One strategy for rationalizing the involvement of pediatricians involved an argument about "seamless webs": promoters of the new-pediatrics emphasized the inseparability of physical and psychosocial problems and the "seamless" nature of a child's well-being. Physical problems that the child might experience, they pointed out (Starfield, 1982:383), could be exacerbated by psychosocial concerns or at least make treatment more complicated. Children with asthma, for example, were more likely than other children to have trouble in school, to be truant, and to be socially isolated. At the same time, children with psychosocial problems were more likely to exhibit physical symptoms, possibly because of the stress associated with psychosocial difficulties. The evidence of a link between stress and disease was abundant in adults. There was no reason to believe that such disease processes played themselves out differently in children. Pediatricians could not purport to care for children's physical well-being without taking the emotional and psychosocial aspects of their development into account.

> There . . . is growing awareness that one cannot, meaningfully fractionate a child's well-being into that which is physical from that which is psychologic and social. The interaction of physical and behavioral development, normal and abnormal, may be complex, but must be acknowledged and understood if truly comprehensive health care is to be provided. (Friedman, 1970:172)

Another strategy involved asserting the continuity between the new pediatrics and the specialty's traditional mission. Even the early proponents of the new pediatrics, for example, pointed out that pediatrics had always been a specialty devoted to the welfare and well-being of children, not just to the treatment and prevention of their diseases. Pediatricians of the past may have concentrated their efforts on disease, they insisted, but only because the high mortality and morbidity rates among children demanded priority. Now that so many physical diseases had been conquered, pediatricians could turn their attention to other problems compromising the well-being of children:

> All science, of which medicine is a major segment is like a multiheaded hydra. Each time one problem is solved, two new ones arise to take its place. Each discovery, while answering some old questions, broadens our horizon so that we constantly see new and more complex problems. . . . The more we learn, the more is seen that we do not understand. (Cole, 1959:642)

They rejected the notion that there was anything *new* about the new pediatrics or about pediatricians adopting a more comprehensive interest in children's lives. The "new pediatrics," they claimed, was a misnomer because the broader view of the pediatrician's role was merely an extension of the specialty's traditional concerns and not a redefinition of its mission in any fundamental sense (Spitz, 1960). The new pediatrics was really only a "shift" (Davison, 1952:536), a natural and logical evolution of the specialty, and an opportunity to practice better pediatrics now that the life-threatening diseases of childhood were out of the way.

In spite of these assertions, the "new pediatrics" persisted as a way of describing pediatricians' more comprehensive interests, emphasizing the ways in which the specialty was changing, and inviting debate over the directions of that change. A new way of talking about pediatricians' concerns was needed.

In 1975, the term "new morbidity" made its way into the pediatric lexicon. The term was coined by Haggerty, Roghmann, and Pless (1975) in their analysis of a series of surveys conducted among families in Monroe County, New York and its main city, Rochester. The purpose of the surveys was to assess the health care needs of preschoolers, school-aged children, and adolescents. The questionnaires tellingly elicited information from parents and teachers about not only the children's physical problems, but their behavioral and school difficulties as well. Mothers of 2 year olds, for example, were asked about behaviors that were causing them concern or worry and leading to frequent conflicts. The most commonly identified behaviors mentioned by the mothers were stubbornness, high activity level and getting into things, temper outbursts, resistance to bedtime, whining, nagging,and demanding attention (Haggerty et al., 1975:97). For school-aged children the question was: "Has he/she ever had trouble with school work; ever been held back a grade; ever been asked to leave school?" The most frequently mentioned "troubles" with schoolwork were academic and reading problems (45%) and behavioral problems such as immaturity, lack of motivation, hyperactivity, and emotional difficulties (35%) (1975:102–103). For adolescents the most common behavioral problems were fighting, restlessness, feeling solitary or withdrawn, and being afraid of things (1975:106).

On the basis of these findings the investigators concluded that

> The major health problems of children today are different from those that prevailed when pediatrics came into existence a century ago. . . . Learning difficulties and school problems, behavioral disturbances, allergies, speech difficulties, visual problems and the problems of adolescents in coping and adjusting are today the most common concerns about children. (Haggerty et al., 1975:316)

They used the term "the new morbidity" to describe these problems. After the mid-1970s, the term gained currency in the profession and increasingly displaced "the new pediatrics."

The significance of the shift lies in the rhetorical effect of the contrasting ways of talking about children's psychosocial difficulties. Haggerty et al. (1975) were not presenting "a point of view" about the appropriate concerns of pediatricians—they were reporting the results of a *scientific* study. They talked not about "the new pediatrics," but about children's "health care needs." And in describing those needs they talked not about "difficulties"—a vague term that begs questions about the nature of those difficulties, but about "morbidity"—a term that assumes their status as illness. Moreover, as "morbidity," there was less question about whether the problems fell within pediatrics' purview.

Haggerty et al. (1975), like other new pediatricians, were making a case for redefining and expanding pediatrics, but they used a scientific rather than a polemic style. The features of a scientific style, as Ibarra and Kitsuse (1993:45) point out, include "a bearing that is disinterested," a tone that is "sober," and a vocabulary that is "technical" and "precise." A scientific style lends an air of objectivity to the assertion being made and diminishes uncertainties about the characterizations proffered.

The effects of a scientific style are demonstrated by Kirk and Kutchins (1992) in their analysis of the American Psychiatric Association's Diagnostic and Statistical Manual of Mental Disorders (DSM). A compendium of mental disorders and their symptoms, the DSM has been described as the "official bible" of the psychiatric profession (Kirk and Kutchins, 1992:2). Kirk and Kutchins (1992) show how it was produced at a time when the very existence of "mental illness" was being questioned and when the general view was that psychiatry did not know what it was talking about. The DSM, by shrouding psychiatric diagnoses in the language and mystique of science, made them more credible. All the diagnostic criteria for the disorders listed in the DSM, Kirk and Kutchins (1992:221) argue, require as much subjectivity and inference as psychiatric diagnoses ever did. But the language used to present these criteria "exudes the spirit of technical rationality." The payoff for psychiatry was a more legitimate and authoritative image. A scientific style does not preclude challenges. Scientists do dispute each other's "findings" or claims (Aronson, 1984; Gillespie and Leffler, 1987). But all the same, it was a more compelling way for the new pediatricians to make their case.

Another subtle but important change in pediatricians' rhetoric around the new pediatrics involved the relationship between pediatrics and child psychiatry. Abbott (1988) speaks about professions as being part of an interdependent system: changes in the jurisdictional boundaries of one profession cannot occur without reverberations throughout the system. Since pediatricians were moving into areas that might be considered the preserve of child psychiatrists, they needed to justify their incursions. Pediatricians initially framed their interest in children's psychosocial problems in terms of the shortage of child psychiatrists (Haggerty, 1982; Hoekelman, 1981; Prugh, 1983:6). Pediatricians needed to take on the task because there were too few child psychiatrists. They exploited the fact that psychiatry in general, and child psychiatry more particularly, had always had recruitment problems. When the Graduate Medical Education National Advisory Council (GMENAC), in 1981, issued its medical manpower projections for 1990, general psychiatry and child psychiatry topped the list of specialties likely to experience a shortage. According to GMENAC, there would be only 4100 child psychiatrists when 9000 would be needed (see Table 4.9). Shortages notwithstanding, some child psychiatrists were disturbed by pediatrics' growing interest in behavioral problems (Anders, 1977; Anders and Niehans, 1982). As one pediatric observer (Haggerty, 1982:393) noted:

> Cynical psychiatrists see behavioral pediatrics as an effort to gain control of the field and its resources. They allege that since pediatrics has solved so many of the acute problems of children, which accounted for their main source of income in the past, they are now forced to look to other fields for income. Since behavioral disturbances are a large problem in the community, pediatricians are seeking to control the market.

"In my experience," he concluded, "this is a minor reason for the emergence of the field."

Gradually pediatricians began to play down the issue of shortages in child psychiatry. They emphasized instead the unique contribution that they could make in alleviating psychosocial and behavioral problems and became clearer about how their services differed from those of child psychiatrists. Pediatricians, they argued, dealt not with the psychopathologies of childhood—with severely depressed children, those who attempted suicide, or had serious run-ins with the law. Serious behavioral disturbances would always remain the terrain of the expertly trained child psychiatrist. Pediatricians were interested in the less serious problems—behaviors that were disruptive, caused conflict, or interfered with the optimal functioning and development of the child, and that, left untreated, might lead to the more serious problems that concerned child psychiatrists.

The shift in rhetoric was in part an effort to placate child psychiatrists who were threatened by the changes in pediatrics and to reassure them that pediatricians had no intention of usurping their traditional areas of practice. But the message was intended for an internal audience as well—those pediatricians who had yet to be convinced that they could make a difference. For these pediatricians, the argument that pediatricians should address children's psychosocial needs because there was not a sufficient number of child psychiatrists to do it was weak, negative, and "unimpressive" (Friedman, 1970:173). Pediatrics' potential contribution needed to be framed in more positive terms.

Proponents of the new pediatrics confidently asserted that pediatricians were uniquely placed to oversee children's development (Reisinger and Bires, 1980) and that even in cases where their concerns overlapped with those of child psychiatrists, pediatricians had qualities that recommended them over child psychiatrists. They were *"the best qualified person the culture has yet provided* to do the liaison job of funneling the new understanding regarding total child care from the Ivory Towers into the stream of child life and family life" (Tompkins, 1959:1015; emphasis added). They had the readiest access to children and their families. They were able to observe children through their formative years and through adolescence.

> As the "general physician" for children, pediatricians are in the most opportune position to monitor the overall growth and development of children, and to intervene where full realization of a child's physical, intellectual and social potential appears in jeopardy. (Friedman, 1970:172)

"More than any other health care provider," the AAP's Committee on Psychosocial Aspects of Child and Family Health argued (AAP, 1982:126), "pediatricians have the requisite longitudinal and cross-sectional perspective, and a background in biologic and psychological development." Moreover, because of the pediatrician's unique position of trust, parents and children alike would feel less threatened by, and more likely to accept, guidance on behavioral matters:

> It should be recognized that the trust and confidence developed between the pediatrician and his patient will often enable him to handle problems more quickly and effectively than the psychiatrist who does not have the advantage of previously established rapport and knowledge of the family. (Yancy, 1975:686)

Finally, the pediatrician's special and on-going relationship with children and their families was used as a basis for contending that whoever else might become involved in the children's care—and pediatricians did allow for the participation of social workers, psychologists, psychotherapists, teachers, guidance counselors, and social scientists—it was the pediatrician who needed to play the central, coordinating role as "head of the team."

CHANGING THE STANDARDS OF CHILD HEALTH CARE

Beyond a carefully reasoned and clearly articulated rationale for expanding pediatrics' scope of practice, proponents of the new pediatrics (or new morbidity) needed to communicate the changing parameters to primary care practitioners. Among the clearest statements of the kind of pediatrics primary care practitioners were now expected to practice were a series of manuals published through the 1960s and 1970s (Hughes, 1980). In 1964, the AAP created a Council on Pediatric Practice, mandating it to "update" the definition of pediatrics in light of the "dramatic and complex changes during the past three decades" (AAP, 1967:i), and to identify desirable standards of practice. By 1967, the Council had produced a manual entitled *Standards of Child Health Care*, which became the AAP's official statement of pediatric's proper scope of practice. The manual, which claimed to present "an outline of the comprehensive health care which should be delivered to children of all ages in health and illness" (AAP, 1967:ii), was updated in 1972 and again in 1977. In the same way that the DSM provides an official map of mental illness and disorder, the successive editions of *Standards of Child Health Care* provide a clear picture of the contours the new pediatrics was slowly taking. Looked at together, they demonstrate the increase in the range of problems subsumed under the new pediatrics and the expansion of the age limits of the specialty. Just as each new edition of the DSM has lengthened the list of behaviors to be treated as mental illness (Kirk and Kutchins, 1992), each new edition of *Standards of Child Health Care* took pediatrics into ever larger spheres of responsibility.

The 1967 edition of *Standards of Child Health Care*, for example, pointed out that pediatricians' responsibilities toward children started not at birth, which tradition had defined as the point at which pediatricians began providing their services, but at conception. It specified as well that pediatrics extended not to 12 years of age, or even 18 years which the AAP had adopted officially as the cut-off age for pediatric patients in 1938 (AAP, 1938), but "through the adolescent years" (AAP, 1967:ii). The 1972 version of the manual set the upper age limit of pediatrics at 21 years.

Between conception and birth, the 1967 manual claimed, pediatricians were to provide any genetic or family planning counseling the family might want or need. Through individual discussion or group conferences, they were to let parents know what to expect, to prepare them for the changes that a new child would bring, to answer their questions, to instill confidence in their natural abilities to care for the child, and to make them aware of community resources they might find helpful. Once the child was born, in addition to looking after the physical needs of the newborn, the pediatrician was to reassure the new mother about the condition of her child, assess her emotional state, provide general instructions in the care of the child, and stress the importance of continuity of pediatric care (AAP, 1967:1–2).

Among the subjects that the manual suggested pediatricians should discuss with parents as the child grew were the dangers of accidents, especially poisonings among young children, the dangers of athletic injuries in older children, feeding techniques, toilet training, the need for, and appropriate methods of discipline, and the value of sex education not only for adolescents but younger children as well. Ideally, the manual clarified, it was up to parents to educate their children on sexual matters, although the pediatrician certainly had a role to play in instructing parents on how to answer their children's questions at various age levels. But if parents found it difficult to cope with the sexual curiosity of their children, the pediatrician should do it.

Interestingly, the manual highlighted the importance of looking beyond those behaviors that might be distressing to parents. The unsophisticated parent, they suggested, might attach importance only to nonconforming behaviors. The alert pediatrician was to watch for excessive conformity, excessive dependence, and a tendency to be "too good" or "too unemotional," traits that could be symptoms of a psychosocial disturbance.

A special section on the treatment of adolescents discussed the need to bring the hazards of smoking, drinking, and drug use to the attention of patients. It encouraged pediatricians to increase the adolescent components of their practices and provided them with advice on how to do so. The manuals hinted that pediatricians needed to find ways to get around their traditional image as a "baby doctor." Youths were likely to assert their growing sense of independence by refusing to see the pediatrician and insisting instead on an "adult doctor." The manual offered suggestions for overcoming the problem. Pediatricians could set up special hours for adolescent patients so that they would not have to share the waiting room with toddlers. They could set up separate examining rooms with less child-oriented and more "dignified" decor. They could satisfy adolescents' desire to be treated like adults by examining them without their parents in the room. This did not mean a diminished role for parents in the traditional doctor–patient relationship in pediatrics. The manuals pointed out that pediatricians should meet with parents before or after the visit to keep them informed.

Finally, the 1967 manual reminded pediatricians that their duties extended beyond their private practices to the community, and that if they did not become involved in child welfare work, other groups would only too willingly fill the void: "Every pediatrician is obligated to the limit of his time and ability, to maintain an active interest in all matters which pertain to the welfare of children in his own community if he does not wish others to assume this role" (AAP, 1967:64). Practising pediatricians should know about the health and welfare agencies and programs in the community. Where facilities were lacking or inadequate, they should foster their establishment or improvement. If laws were inadequate, as, for example, in the case of adoptions, pediatric societies should cooperate with bar associations to change them.

The 1972 version of the manual identified more precisely the problems pediatricians might confront in providing emotional or anticipatory guidance, and specified in more inclusive terms the role that pediatricians should play in managing these problems. The list was exhaustive. It included not only children's misbehaviors but parental difficulties as well: maternal insecurity with the child, reactions to congenital malformations, crying, the working mother and her feelings of guilt, fatigue, the adopted child, the hyperactive child, the mentally retarded child, the gifted child, the whiny child, tempers, deviations in appetite, jealousy, disobedience, selfishness, lying, parental fears, fear of lightning, the dark, animals and peers, destructiveness, enuresis (bed wetting), stealing, fighting with siblings and peers, bullying, inability to make friends, overconformity, being too tall, short, thin, or heavy, setting fires, inattention at home or school, underachievement at school, parental overprotection, parental rejection of the child, acceptance of gender (boys acting in a feminine manner, tomboys), depression, alcoholism in parents, family discord, divorce and the child, adolescence (the struggle for independence, sexual adjustment, obtaining jobs, drug use and smoking), and sex education.

The pediatrician could bring most of these problems to light, the 1972 manual noted (AAP, 1972), with a few routine questions. Its appendices included a behavior questionnaire for preschoolers that pediatricians could have mothers fill out prior to the well-child interviews. As far as their management was concerned, the manual suggested that pediatricians might find it useful to refer the child to other experts, but added: "The problems usually will not warrant psychiatric referral but can be handled adequately by a pediatrician. Consequently, the pediatrician should prepare himself to handle many of these problems. . . . He should be prepared to discuss these problems with parents and to give advice and counsel" (AAP, 1972:14).

Another feature of the 1972 manual was its discussion of sex education in various age groups. Reacting to a public backlash against sex education in schools, it affirmed the AAP's commitment to sex education programs not only in schools but churches and other community institutions. Pediatricians were encouraged to use their professional authority and standing in the community to convert a resistant public to the merits of family life and sex education programs:

> Pediatricians, with their position of acceptance and trust in the community, have an unusual opportunity and a responsibility to add their voices

in support and direction of the family life and sex education programs. Every effort must be made to work through parents, support public school officials, and join in sponsoring and participating in public meetings which discuss the content and goals of sex education and family life programs. (AAP, 1972:17)

The updated discussion of family planning in the 1972 manual added population control to the pediatrician's already long list of professional duties. Pediatricians, it stated, should be aware of the social, health, and demographic problems associated with prolific child bearing and should work with parents and teachers to give young people a proper sense of responsibility about sexual matters, marriage, and parenthood. Pediatricians should provide information and advice about contraception to sexually active adolescents and counseling for unwed mothers.

The 1977 revision of the manual went further still, including for the first time the ethical development of children as part of the pediatric mandate. The manual argued that it was natural for parents to turn to pediatricians with questions about the fundamental moral and religious values they should instill in their children. Pediatricians, as respected members of their communities, had a duty to provide that assistance:

In a time when social issues and conflict are part of daily life, the doctor can make a meaningful contribution to the education of children and parents by sharing himself in these ways. This dimension of a child's growth is a legitimate and valued part of pediatric practice. (AAP, 1977:30–31)

There were several ways pediatricians might "share themselves." They could act as role models, demonstrating dedication, integrity, understanding, and caring; as facilitators, helping families explore and identify problem areas and seek their own values, as counselors, offering advice on specific issues; and as bridging agents, weighing for their patients both the values and limitations of traditional views of good and evil in the context of contemporary society.

The definition of pediatrics presented in *Standards of Child Health Care* was reinforced at professional meetings, workshops, seminars, and roundtables, and through a broad range of materials that became available to primary care pediatricians. These materials included pamphlets, audiotapes, testing and assessment schedules, and detailed packets for health supervision visits covering every age category from the prenatal period to adolescence. The message was categorical: unless primary care practitioners were prepared to understand health in the broadest possible terms and to meet the challenge of attending to their patients' total health care needs, they were failing to live up to their professional responsibilities as pediatricians.

EDUCATIONAL REFORM

While pediatric organizations, especially the AAP, promoted the image of a more comprehensive pediatrics to establish the new pediatrics as the standard of practice, pediatric training programs remained basically unchanged through the 1960 and 1970s. Though a few pediatric departments tried to make their programs more responsive to primary care pediatricians by preparing them to take on the psychosocial and behavioral problems they were likely to confront and expected to treat in their practices, most of the academic community continued to resist any alteration to the science- and disease-based curricula. Primary care pediatricians were left in an impossible situation. They were exhorted by the specialty's leaders to broaden their scope of practice, but they received little or no training in the new problems they were supposed to treat. The more firmly organized pediatrics committed the specialty to the new morbidity in pediatrics, the more obvious and problematic the paradox became and the greater the pressure on the academic community to introduce changes.

Through 1973 and 1974 an angry exchange heated the pages of *Pediatrics*. The debate began when David G. Nathan, chief of the Division of Hemotology–Oncology at Boston's Children's Hospital Medical Center, wrote a commentary on an address given by Cicely Williams to the hospital's alumni association in May 1973. Williams had admonished pediatric academics for their misplaced emphasis on disease and for not incorporating more of the concerns of primary care pediatricians into their training programs:

> Be off with your ultrascience, your superspecialists and your rapt attention to the few with so called interesting illnesses. Give thought instead to the thousands who are sick because of neglect at home. Free them from malnutrition of the body or the soul, and society will reap immediate benefits. Teachers, stop seducing the very best into your snare of enzymes, isotopes and transducers, leaving only a small group to replace our dwindling cohort of primary care deliverers. If you will only see the challenge of home care and preventive care, the bright ones will follow you there. (Williams, 1973:773)

Nathan was sympathetic to Williams' argument that pediatric educators needed to pay more attention to preparing students for careers in primary care practices. Williams' message, he stated, "should be carefully studied by all pediatricians, and particularly by pediatricians involved in academic programs" (Nathan, 1973:768). He conceded that "we have encouraged the cream to rise to the top, the top defined as

specialty and research medicine, without due regard for the overall benefits to society of such a policy" (1973:769). Nathan recognized as well
that preparing pediatricians for primary care meant that pediatric programs would need to add an entirely different subject matter to the
curriculum, courses in public health procedures, medical economics,
basic sociologic principles, and the interactions of government and
society.

But he pleaded that training for primary care not occur at the expense
of a solid background in the diseases of children. Whatever attention the
developmental and psychosocial problems of children got, he argued, it
should be a supplement to, and not a replacement for, the emphasis in
the curriculum on the physical problems of children. Without a scientific
grounding in the treatment of disease, according to Nathan, the practice
of medicine would revert to the "gold-headed cane era when personality
was in fact the only tool of the trade" (1973:770).

But the "piece de resistance," as a fellow pediatrician (Shiller,
1974:131) later put it, was Nathan's proposal that it should be "senior"
academics, those with an established record in the diseases of children,
who should provide the training in primary care. The best and the
brightest of pediatrics' young academics were to be reserved for serious
scientific research and teaching. Younger academics did not have the
time to retrain themselves in the new pediatrics. "They need more than
24 hours a day," he wrote (Nathan, 1973:771), "to solve the biomedical
problems that confront them." Those pediatricians who had already
made their contributions to science, on the other hand, and were no
longer "excited by laboratory investigations," might find the challenge
appealing. Moreover, Nathan insisted that these older academics had
the perspective and research skills that might prove useful in developing
a knowledge base for the new pediatrics. The implication was that they
would bring a degree of scientific rigor that the new pediatrics currently
lacked. "I somehow feel very comfortable," he continued (1973:772),
"when I see a man who is capable of precise measurement of the rate at
which potassium enters a red cell, applying the same sort of thinking to
an estimate of the rate and extent to which primary care physicians must
be deployed in the city of New York." His recommendation, Nathan
concluded, would meet two objectives: it would keep those young and
recently trained minds "at the helm" in research and it would provide
new challenges for older investigators who had "the tough crust and the
experience to plunge into icy waters" (1973:771). Nowhere in his commentary did Nathan consider the possibility of bringing in academically
oriented clinicians—pediatricians with years of experience and a strong
commitment to a comprehensive pediatrics at the primary care level—to
teach new recruits.

Nathan's remarks sparked a storm of outraged protest. He was criticized for his condescension and "intellectual elitism" (Pyeritz, 1974:249).
"Dr. Nathan's naivete with respect to problems outside the hematology
laboratory," wrote one pediatrician (Katcher, 1974:251), "is matched only
by his arrogance." Michael K. Posner (1974:249), medical director of the
Woodlawn Child Health Center in Chicago, ridiculed the suggestion
that aging academics should be the ones to develop programs in primary
care pediatrics. "In no other area of investigation would a researcher
suggest that a particularly vexing problem be tackled by those no longer
productive in the areas of their choice." It was these "grand old men"
who had created the problem in the first place, he argued, by emphasizing scientific medicine at the expense of total patient care. Posner and
many others who responded to Nathan's views (Bass et al., 1974; Katcher, 1974; Pyeritz, 1974; Shiller, 1974) maintained that it should be
academically oriented pediatric practitioners, not a "few research war-
horses sent out to the primary care pasture" (Posner, 1974:249), who
should teach primary care pediatrics.

Nathan's solution to the problems that existed in pediatric education,
in the form of reschooling for older investigators in the social sciences
relevant to primary care, may have been novel. But the underlying attitude about the place of psychosocial problems vis-à-vis the physical
problems of children, and the significance of primary care vis-à-vis the
scientific components of pediatric training, were not. Most academics,
like Nathan, felt strongly about maintaining the scientific direction of
training and were reluctant to make space available in the pediatric
curricula for primary care or general pediatrics and behavioral, psychosocial, and developmental problems.

Not surprising, studies through the 1970s showed that pediatricians
felt ill-prepared to deal with problems in these areas. In a survey of 61
pediatricians in South Florida (Toister and Worley, 1976), for example,
89% of respondents stated that more than 10% of their daily calls or
office visits involved specific requests for behavioral information or
guidance. More than half of the respondents reported that they had
insufficient training or no training at all to help them deal with these
problems. Seventy-nine percent of 97 randomly selected pediatricians in
five New England states stated that their formal training in developmental pediatrics was inadequate (Dworkin et al., 1979). Although 99% felt
that their clinical experience was a valuable source of information about
children with educational, emotional, and other developmental problems, almost two-thirds did not regard it as an adequate substitute for
formal training.

Several factors converged through the 1970s to force changes in pediatric education. Most critical was the report of the Task Force on Pediatric

Education. In 1976, 10 organizations (AAP, APS, ABP, SPR, Ambulatory
Pediatrics Association, Association of Pediatric Chairmen, AMA Residency Review Committee, Society of Adolescent Medicine, Academy of
Child Psychiatry, and Professors of Child Psychiatry) formed a 17-mem-
ber Task Force to "identify the health needs of infants, children and
adolescents" and "to point out the educational strategies that are required to prepare pediatricians of the future to meet them" (Kempe,
1978:1150). The Task Force met monthly for 2 years. It commissioned a
survey of doctors who had graduated from pediatric residency programs
since 1964. The survey results were consistent with other studies on
how graduates felt about their training. They showed that 80% of pediatricians were being asked to provide services such as counseling and
management of learning disorders and other psychosocial problems.
They showed, as well, that a majority—54%—viewed their residency
training in these areas as inadequate (Table 5.1). Sixty-six percent felt ill-
equipped in adolescent medicine, 41% in interviewing and counseling,
64% in school health, 73% in community programs such as nursery

Table 5.1.   Pediatricians' Evaluations of Pediatric Residency Training

Areas of Care	Insufficient (%)	Sufficient (%)	Excessive (%)	N/A (%)
Longitudinal care of well children as opposed to episodic care	50.4	48.4	0.5	0.6
Care of adolescents	65.9	33.0	0.3	0.8
Care of children with chronic physical dysfunction	18.4	74.2	7.0	0.6
Care of children with chronic cerebral dysfunction	40.4	56.8	2.1	0.6
Psychosocial and/or behavioral problems	53.9	44.1	1.2	0.8
Interviewing and counseling	40.8	57.1	1.3	0.8
Ambulatory care within the medical school hospital	11.4	79.9	7.1	1.6
Ambulatory care in an extramural setting	44.8	49.6	1.9	3.7
Preparation for involvement in child advocacy (the poor, racial minorities, single-parented children, abused and handicapped children)	50.5	46.8	2.1	0.8
School health	64.3	34.7	0.3	0.7
Community programs (custodial institutions, juvenile courts, programs for exceptional children)	73.1	26.1	0.3	0.5

Source: Task Force on Pediatric Education (1978:7).

schools, juvenile courts, custodial institutions for young people, and programs for exceptions children, and 50% in child advocacy related to child abuse, neglect, and mental retardation (Task Force on Pediatric Education, 1978).

The report that the Task Force ultimately released in 1978 concluded that pediatric training was woefully inadequate to meet the needs of most pediatricians, and that the grossest deficits were in precisely those areas that represented what the committee considered the "bases of the specialty"—the biosocial and developmental aspects of pediatrics. The other most significantly underemphasized area, according to the Task Force, was adolescence. "The health needs of adolescents," it noted, "are being inadequately met. Pediatrics should now take upon itself the full responsibility for improving health care and research for this segment of the American population" (1978:22). Other areas singled out by the Task Force were community pediatrics, the care of children with handicaps and chronic conditions, health promotion, nutrition, medical ethics, and child advocacy.

C. Henry Kempe, the Task Force chairman, and at the time president of the APS, commented after the report was published on how frustrating and annoying he had found the attitudes of many pediatric program directors: "The concept that educational activities in our departments should relate to the health needs of children was not as universally accepted as you might think," he complained. "A few feel to this day that it should be the other way round, that the needs of their departments should be addressed by a ready supply of sick and funded children, each in their appropriate subspecialty" (Kempe, 1978:1150). He suggested that "instead of moaning about whether our residents are being overtrained for what they do," program directors should "face the fact that they are undertrained for what they are being asked to do" (Kempe, 1978:1151).

The Task Force report recommended a much greater stress on ambulatory care and the new morbidity in pediatrics, the behavioral problems of preschoolers, inadequate functioning in schools, and problems related to adolescence. "The health needs of children and adolescents should be explicitly considered in planning educational programs" (Task Force on Pediatric Education, 1978:x). "There should be increased emphasis on the biosocial aspects of pediatrics and adolescent health." In a more general vein the report asserted that

The purpose of the educational process is to prepare pediatricians to provide comprehensive and continuing care which will meet the health needs of infants, children and adolescents. Pediatricians must be increasingly concerned with the quality of their patients' lives and with fostering the opportunity for each child to become an intact adult—physically, psychologically and socially. (Task Force on Pediatric Education, 1978:10)

Comprehensive pediatrics was defined in terms at least as broad as those used in the AAP's *Standards of Child Health Care*:

> Residents should learn to manage such family crises as death and bereavement, suicide attempts, sexual assaults, accidents, child abuse, birth of a defective child, separation, divorce, abortion, and a wide range of behavioral disorders. Furthermore, they should be able to work with the family to resolve problems in parenting, well-child care, adoption/foster care, school management and learning. (Task Force on Pediatric Education, 1978:22)

To allow sufficient time for these issues to be covered in pediatric training, the Task Force recommended that the period of training in general pediatrics that residents were required to undergo before entering practice or subspecializing be extended from 2 to 3 years. In 1978, the Pediatric Residency Review Committee, which prepares guidelines for residency programs, for the first time mandated a 3-year residency for pediatrics, identified a "commitment to primary care," and recommended 6 months of ambulatory experience for all residents. In 1982 the ABP accepted the recommendation of the Task Force making 3 years of core pediatric training a condition for licensure. The ABP also appointed a subcommittee to develop test items on biosocial and behavioral pediatrics for incorporation into the board's written and oral examinations.

While the Task Force on Education created the pressure to reform, groups outside pediatrics provided financial incentives. During the late 1970s, two foundations, the Robert Wood Johnson Foundation and the W. T. Grant Foundation, and the U.S. Bureau of Health Manpower all began sponsoring training in general and behavioral pediatrics. The Robert Wood Johnson Foundation supported improvements in health services, particularly among underserviced segments of the population. In 1973, it began funding demonstration programs in primary care pediatrics and internal medicine at nine medical schools. The objective was to develop models for other programs to follow in the training of doctors who intended to practice general medicine within their respective age ranges. Though the programs differed markedly in their approaches, they all emphasized ambulatory care, and in particular continuous and comprehensive patient care (Rosinski and Dagenais, 1978).

Another six pediatric programs in general pediatrics received funding in 1975 from the U.S. Bureau of Health Manpower. The Bureau had been lobbying for government support for primary care training in pediatrics, internal medicine and family medicine. Its intention in awarding the six grants was to ensure that once the money was allocated, there would be a model for funded programs to follow. In 1976, the U.S. Congress passed the Health Professions Educational Assistance Act, which made it possible for the 15 programs initially sponsored by the Robert Wood Johnson Foundation and the Bureau of Health Manpower to continue. It also allowed for the establishment of another 36 programs in general pediatrics.

The W. T. Grant Foundation had a more focused mandate. It supported research, professional training, and social policy and advocacy projects concerned specifically with the psychological and social development of children and youth. In 1978, the Foundation offered training grants to medical schools interested in integrating behavioral pediatrics into their residency programs for pediatricians. The Foundation awarded a total of two million dollars to 11 programs. In 1981, the foundation renewed the grants at a cost of another two million dollars.

The financial support that these groups provided was significant in the process of educational reform in pediatrics in two respects. In a concrete sense, the funding covered the expenses involved in restructuring training programs, for those medical schools that received the grants. More importantly, the funding signaled to all pediatric departments that the movement toward the new pediatrics within the specialty had the support of government and key policymakers who were determined to see pediatricians provide more comprehensive primary care to children.

Educational reform was facilitated as well by the availability of pediatric educators trained and qualified to teach the new pediatrics. A substantial deterrent to reform in the past had been pediatrics' reliance on child psychiatrists. Those programs that had established liaisons with child psychiatry had not found the arrangement entirely satisfactory. Child psychiatrists had difficulty communicating with pediatric residents. Pediatricians, it seemed, were too problem oriented to get much out of the insights of psychiatry. They found child psychiatry "rich in theory," but "short on empirical observations" (Richmond, 1967:652). Leon Eisenberg, a child psychiatrist at the Johns Hopkins Hospital who participated in a pediatric-child psychiatry liaison program, admitted that child psychiatry was too abstract and esoteric for pediatricians: "Pediatricians, with their grounding in laboriously acquired empirical data, controlled therapeutic trials and action-oriented methods of intervention, find it difficult to swallow . . . the untestable theories, the talmudical disputation based on an appeal to authority" (Eisenberg, 1967:645). The need for long hours of analysis and assessment that were the child psychiatrist's "tools of the trade" did not fit well with pediatrics' economics of practice. Pediatricians could not afford to spend long periods of time with patients. And, finally, there were concerns about bringing in "outsiders" to train pediatricians and relinquishing control over part of the pediatric curriculum. Child psychiatrists and pediatricians alike agreed that "the teachers of pediatricians must be pediatricians" (Eisenberg, 1967:645).

The fellowship programs that had been set up in behavioral and developmental areas of pediatrics during the late 1960s and 1970s, however, had produced a "new breed" (Richmond, 1975:521) of pediatrician—pediatricians dedicated exclusively to studying and treating these aspects of children's health and to providing quality health care to adolescents. As pediatric departments responded to the Task Force Report by initiating reform in their programs, there was an "in-house" corps of pediatricians ready, eager, and willing to introduce their colleagues to the new pediatrics.

Moreover, these specialized pediatricians were already beginning to develop conceptual frameworks and practical techniques for dealing with behavioral and psychosocial problems that were better suited to pediatricians than the approaches taken by psychiatry. Rather than aiming for the reflective, deeper understanding of the meaning of seriously aberrant behaviors, acquired over long hours of analysis and assessment, they concentrated on early intervention, the quick relief of symptoms, and the treatment of less severe problems using advice-giving and behavioral counseling (Richmond, 1975:522). Their more functional, practical, and problem-oriented approaches fit well with pediatricians' style of practice.

Chapter 6

Assessing the New Pediatrics

Over the past three decades those who envisioned a more comprehensive pediatrics with broad-ranging responsibility for children's total health care needs have come a long way in making that vision a reality. The new pediatrics is no longer simply a blueprint for the specialty's future but a more or less accurate description of what pediatrics has become. Those who have chosen behavioral or developmental pediatrics, adolescent medicine, and general pediatrics as areas of academic subspecialization have done particularly well. Once on the margins of academic life, they have become vital, productive members of pediatric training programs (Haggerty, 1990). Besides their own organizations, they have their own journals (*the Journal of Behavioral and Developmental Pediatrics* and the *Journal of Adolescent Health Care*). They publish prolifically not only in these journals but in mainstream pediatric and medical journals as well. There has been a virtual explosion over the past two decades in papers, textbooks, monographs, and book chapters providing both general overviews of behavioral and adolescent health care concerns and more detailed treatments of specific problems (Richmond and Janis, 1983:21–22). The specialized knowledge base that is essential to the further development of the new pediatrics (Haggerty, 1988) is rapidly being built. Whatever may happen at the level of primary care pediatrics then, behavioral pediatrics, adolescent medicine, and perhaps even general pediatrics are likely to survive as academic subspecialties.

But not all the issues around the new pediatrics have been resolved. The success of academics in the area notwithstanding, pediatric education continues to be an issue for the specialty. The first evaluations of pediatric training after the Task Force on Pediatric Education (1978) published its report were not encouraging. A survey of 29 pediatric programs, conducted in 1983, 5 years after the Task Force report was issued, indicated that though there had been an increase in the number of courses offered in areas subsumed under the new pediatrics, the increase was not dramatic (Table 6.1). The number of programs offering training in continuous care increased from 19 in 1978 to 25 in 1983, in child development from 19 to 20, in behavioral pediatrics from 16 to 20,

Table 6.1. Number of Elective and Mandatory Programs in the New Morbidity

	Elective		Mandatory	
	Before 1978	After 1978	Before 1978	After 1978
Continuity of care	3	1	16	24
Child development	8	7	11	13
Child psychiatry/behavioral pediatrics	10	7	6	13
Adolescent medicine	4	8	12	14
Handicapping condition	8	9	7	9
Ethics	—	2	1	1
Genetic counseling	8	13	3	6
Extramural primary care	13	15	5	9

Source: Weinberger and Oski (1984:525).

in adolescent medicine from 16 to 22, in handicapping conditions from 15 to 18, in genetic counseling from 11 to 19, and in extramural primary care from 18 to 24.

The same survey showed that in a sizable number of programs, many courses in the new morbidity were still elective rather than mandatory, an arrangement that advocates of the new pediatrics argue is a convenient "copout" for programs that were ambivalent about the value of the new pediatrics (Table 6.1). The ratio of elective to mandatory courses in child development was 7:13, in behavioral pediatrics 7:13, in adolescent medicine 8:14, in handicapping conditions 9:9, in genetic counseling 13:6, and in extramural primary care 15:9.

A comparison of the actual content of pediatric training, in terms of the total time residents spend in different areas of pediatrics, revealed even more clearly how little things had changed (Table 6.2). There was virtually no difference in the percentage of time that residents prior to 1978 and those after 1978 spend in mandatory disease-oriented areas

Table 6.2. Total Time Spent During 3-Year Residency

	Before 1978		After 1978	
	Months	Percent	Months	Percent
Inpatient	12.1	34	12.0	34
Outpatient	7.7	22	7.2	21
Neonatal	6.3	18	5.9	17
Subspecialty	3.4	10	3.3	10
Electives	6.2	17	6.5	18

Source: Weinberger and Oski (1984:525).

such as inpatient care (34 vs. 34%), neonatal medicine (18 vs. 17%), and subspecialty care (10 vs. 10%). The percentage of time devoted to outpatient care actually dropped slightly from 22% in 1978 to 21% in 1983.

Another problem that behaviorally oriented pediatricians complained about was the low priority that some faculty and students alike attached to the outpatient aspects of their training. Friedman, Phillips, and Parrish (1983) observed in an on-site review of the model programs funded by the W. T. Grant Foundation, that few programs attempted to deal seriously with this problem. In only two out of the eight programs that incorporated training in the new pediatrics into their outpatient clinics did the programs make clear that it expected students to attend regularly and to treat it with the same degree of seriousness and commitment they brought to other aspects of their training. In those two departments, students were actually called if they were absent.

More recent surveys appear at first glance to be more positive. Mathieu and Alpert (1987) found that 90% of pediatric residency programs included curricula in developmental and behavioral pediatrics. Though the figure is an improvement over previous findings, Mathieu and Alpert stress that they found considerable ambivalence, if not tension, regarding training for general, primary care pediatrics. Most leaders in academic medicine are still subspecialists in organically based areas of pediatrics and continue to emphasize traditional concerns. Others (Charney, 1995:270) have described the ambivalence as "a kind of schizophrenia that exists about primary care education within traditional pediatrics . . . a split allegiance to consultative and primary medicine." According to Charney (1995), though many pediatric departments verbalize the importance of primary care programs for their trainees, their efforts remain invested "on the ward." Charney's (1995:271) final assessment is that despite the incremental gains and pediatrics' steadfast commitment to primary care, "the issues of 20 years ago are still with us." Other long-time observers of pediatric education (Alpert, 1991:188) agree that pediatrics has yet to "get its educational house in order."

The slow and disappointing pace of change in training programs suggests that although pediatric academics may be complying with the letter of the Task Force recommendations concerning the new pediatrics, they have not wholeheartedly espoused the spirit and still have doubts about the course the profession has chosen to follow. Indeed, many academics have publicly stated as much, echoing many of the complaints that Charles May voiced (Chapter 3) in the 1960s when pediatrics first began venturing into new areas of care. They feel that the primary care of children does not require the input of highly trained specialists like pediatricians. Much of it, especially the treatment of behavioral and developmental problems, could be handled more effectively and more inexpensively by groups such as family practitioners and PNPs (Davis, 1975:840). They feel the behavioral aspects of the new pediatrics are "too soft" to be academically respectable and continue to worry that pediatrics will lose its appeal to medical students if the focus in training turns too much away from the sick child.

> The emphasis on primary care, with its heavy emphasis on the psychosocial aspects (better provided by other than physicians) may turn many of the very bright, currently graduating medical students away from pediatrics as a career. Those particularly interested in this aspect may, as they already have, turn instead to family practice. Recruitment of highly capable physicians into pediatrics may become difficult. (Cleveland, 1985:910)

They worry that too strong an emphasis on the new morbidity in training may undermine the ability of general pediatricians to perform the medical aspects of their job, so that when they come across children with diabetes mellitus, heart murmurs, or seizures—conditions that they feel a well-trained pediatrician should be able to evaluate and manage on their own—they refer them to subspecialists:

> We are physicians first of all, and I fear that overemphasis on the psychosocial aspects of care may have weakened our capability to perform our primary task: the medical care of sick children. We can be expert in child development without becoming psychologists, sensitive to the psychosocial needs of patients and families without becoming social workers and prompt in discovering educational problems without becoming educators. (Garfunkel, 1985:911)

Finally, they continue to question the specialty's motives for insisting so vigorously on a place in primary care:

> The current popular support for continuing the role of the pediatrician as a provider of primary care derives to some extent from the reliance of practising pediatricians on this activity as their major source of financial support. This has been clearly stated by some pediatricians. However understandable, this should not justify the continuance of a system if it is not best in the long run. (Cleveland, 1985:910)

Many academicians candidly admit that they prefer to see pediatrics move out of primary care, and back toward a consulting model of care.

> Our own training program has responded to the current emphasis on primary care, and will continue to do so as long as this is the policy chosen by organized pediatrics. My personal convictions are, however, that this is the wrong direction for the long haul and that the needs of children will be

best served by a gradual orientation toward use of the pediatrician as a consultant. (Cleveland, 1985:911)

As they see it, a certain number of pediatricians would be needed as consultants in general pediatrics, filling the gap between primary care physicians and subspecialists. They would take on more of the physical problems that pediatricians currently tend to refer to subspecialists, freeing the subspecialists to spend more time on research and less on clinical care of children. They would also take on those complex cases that fall between the subspecialty cracks. And they would assist in the training of family and nurse practitioners and students. But the majority of pediatricians would have to move into other areas of medicine—public health or perhaps administrative positions (Garfunkel, 1985).

The persistent ambivalence of the academic community is reflected among practitioners who are reluctant to embrace the new pediatrics. The most recent studies here indicate that primary care pediatricians are still "missing" much of the new morbidity that passes through their offices and clinics. In one study (Costello et al., 1988) primary care practitioners diagnosed the presence of emotional and behavioral problems in 5.6% of children. This figure represented only 17% of children who actually had emotional or behavioral problems as ascertained in an independent psychiatric assessments of the children. The authors concluded that "there is still some way to go before the magnitude of the new morbidity is fully recognized" (Costello et al., 1988:424). They suggest that the new morbidity is still the "hidden morbidity."

More positively, another study (Sharp et al., 1992) shows that in a majority of child health supervision visits (88%), parents and children are being given the opportunity to express their psychosocial concerns and do, frequently mentioning such problems as insecurity, trouble in interpersonal relationships, and learning difficulties. The authors interpreted the finding as a reflection of the increased training in these issues. Primary care pediatricians seem to be aware that the goal of the child health supervision visit is to gather information about the psychosocial problems of children and their families. But they are still slow to provide guidance in these areas. In only 40% of cases did the physicians respond with information, reassurance, guidance, or referral. In 17% of the cases physicians ignored the concern and in 43%, although they asked exploratory questions and elicited more information, they provided no information, reassurance or guidance. Sharp et al. (1992:622) cite a case where the physician had successfully established rapport with both mother and child and had asked the mother in an open and nonjudgmental way, "Do you have any concerns?" The mother responded emphatically and, according to the authors, with considerable affect:

"Yes, her behavior!" at which point the 7-year-old girl emphasized the point by pulling the doctor's tie. His next question was: "So she's been pretty healthy, no fevers or anything since the last visit?" The mother kept returning to the issue of her child's behavioral problems and her difficulty in getting along with other children at school, but got no response. Sharp et al. (1992) conclude that the new morbidity is not so much "hidden" as it is "unheeded."

On a humorous, but no less graphic note, the new pediatrics has occasionally become the object of ridicule in the pediatric literature. Bothered by their lack of athletic prowess, Burke and McGee (1990) recently identified an undescribed illness called Sports Deficit Disorder, the symptoms of which include (1) always being the last one to get to play, and then only when the game is hopelessly lost or definitely won; (2) always being made to play right field; (3) never having dated a cheerleader; (4) being able to describe all your athletic highpoints in less than 10 words; and (5) having hand callouses developed by holding blocking dummies, or body bruises developed by being a blocking dummy. The treatment Burke and McGee suggest is methylphenidate (Ritalin) to block out distracting stimuli and thus fulfill the coach's admonition to "keep your eye on the ball" and stanazolol, an anabolic steroid, to "take the pitcher downtown" whenever he does hit the ball. "We appeal to our fellow physicians," Burke and McGee (1990:1118) write, "to be alert for this new and devastating pediatric disorder. Once these children and their parents understand that it is not the child's fault that he is athletically inept, but rather that he suffers from a definite disease, then we feel that progress can be made to restore the child's damaged self-image." A colleague (Crook, 1990:804) responded:

> Although they wrote their delightful commentary "tongue in cheek," in my opinion, labeling other children with the diagnosis "attention deficit disorder" and prescribing Ritalin may also need to be ridiculed.

In the area of adolescent care, pediatricians have virtually ceded the adolescent population to family practitioners (Budetti, Frey, and McManus, 1982; Nadler and Evans, 1987:25). Those who want to see adolescent medicine integrated within general pediatrics have complained that too many residents consider adolescent medicine to be outside the mainstream of the specialty and that primary care pediatricians too often send problem adolescents elsewhere for care. Zack (1981:733) describes adolescent medicine as "an outcast"—"a forsaken member of the family of pediatrics." Successes notwithstanding, then, the transformation of the pediatrics from the old to the new remains incomplete.

THE FUTURE FOR PRIMARY CARE PEDIATRICS

How much of the new morbidity pediatricians ultimately take on is a question over which pediatrics has at least some control. The future of the specialty will be influenced as well, however, by those same factors that have had such a profound effect on its past and over which pediatricians have less control—the demographics of the child population and developments among other child health care providers. The numbers are not encouraging. Birth rates rose slightly through the late 1970s and 1980s as women of the baby boom generation have moved through their child bearing years. But the birth rate peaked at 16.7 per 1000 population in 1990 and is now declining. The figures for 1992 and 1993 were 16 and 15.7, respectively (Wegman, 1994). The U.S. Bureau of the Census projects that the size of the younger than 20-year-old population will grow until the year 2000, after which the size of the population is expected to stabilize at 72–73 million until the year 2050 (AMA Council on Long Range Planning and Development, 1987:242).

Matched against the likely growth in the number of pediatricians, the ratio of children to pediatricians will also probably decline. The AMA's Council on Long Range Planning and Development (1987:242), a group that studies trends in the environment of medicine and identifies the implications for physicians, estimates that the number of children per pediatrician will decline from 3098 in 1970 to 1254 in 2000. In other words, the Council predicts a ratio of less than half as many children per pediatrician for the year 2000 compared with 1970.

A recent update of the manpower projections prepared by the Graduate Medical Education National Advisory Council (GMENAC) is another source of concern. The figures show that the projected surplus for 1990 should have been 7289, not 4950 as the 1980 GMENAC committee had originally predicted (Eaton, 1991). The surplus projected for the year 2000 is 12,931, and for 2010, 18,462. Again, pediatricians have challenged the numbers arguing:

> The Academy and the nation must address critical policy problems regarding pediatric manpower—maldistribution, underrepresented minorities and the development of adequate numbers of pediatricians to care for children who currently are uninsured or underinsured. But an oversupply of pediatricians is not one of them. (Eaton, 1991:871)

Pediatricians are resisting any effort to limit the training of more pediatricians. Testifying before the Council on Graduate Medical Education, a group asked to advise congress on the supply and distribution of physicians, the AAP and several pediatric research societies insisted that "the current number of pediatric residents be maintained until data are found to substantiate the need for either an increase or decrease in the number of residents based on changes in children's health care needs" (Council on Graduate Medical Education, 1988:23). They insist that any curtailment of primary care pediatrics would be shortsighted:

> Pediatrics is not dying; it still offers the best opportunity among the clinical disciplines to affect individuals at a time in their lives when intervention counts, when disease can be totally averted or minimized. This aspect of pediatrics has always been appealing to a segment of our students and the discipline and its practitioners should show it, in all of its appeal, to those students. The time for platitudes (and worry) is past; the time for action is here. (Fulginiti, 1987:248)

Exacerbating trends indicating an oversupply of pediatricians is the continuing competition from other child health care providers. Family practice has grown, in the words of one pediatrician (Charney, 1995:270) from "a frail newborn to a lusty adolescent." Thirteen percent of all American medical school graduates opted for family practice residencies in 1994, the highest percentage in a decade. Due largely to the AAP's aggressive promotional campaigns, pediatricians have made advances relative to general/family practitioners in the percentage of office visits for various child age categories. With the prospect of even more intense competition between the two specialties, the AMA Council of Long Range Planning and Development (1987:243) speculates that general/family practitioners may decide to concentrate on other, growing parts of the population, such as the elderly, rather than competing directly with pediatricians for children. But there is no indication yet that family practitioners are prepared to abdicate their place in the child health care market. On the contrary, younger family practitioners, in contrast to those who are closer to retirement, are more likely to try to increase the child health care component of their practices (Budetti et al., 1982). In the view of some pediatricians, the "turf battles [between pediatricians and family practitioners] undoubtedly will continue" (Haggerty, 1995:811).

With respect to PNPs, the AAP recently endorsed the role of PNPs, but only in an interdependent relationship [with pediatricians] . . . and a clear understanding between both parties of the roles of each" (AAP, 1994:22). The AAP insists that pediatricians "supervise" the work of PNPs. Given the continued animosity between pediatricians and PNPs, the AMA Council on Long Range Planning and Development (1987:243) observes that "the professional niche of PNPs has eroded in the current socioeconomic environment . . . and is not likely to reemerge." But the

Council also contemplates the possibility that PNPs may seek a competitive role as either independent providers of services for children or as employees in alternative delivery systems. On this score, the Council may be right. Loretta Ford (1982:245), the cofounder of the country's first PNP program, has urged her colleagues "to develop [their] personal, institutional and professional organizational strategies to create an active (rather than reactive), funded, and well-oiled political machine." She recommends the preparation of special nurses for "statesmanship." These nurses would fight the political battles for legislative recognition, reimbursement, and educational funding. They would also pursue "new and creative partnerships" with consumers and local community groups.

Other leaders of the nurse practitioner movement concur that the best hope for the movement is to bypass the medical profession and traditional practice environments (primary care clinics, physicians' offices, and health maintenance organizations) and to look for practice opportunities that offer more autonomy and independence, and that are not "overrun with physicians" (Billingsley and Harper, 1982:30). Billingsley and Harper argue that

> The move toward new practice territory is essential if we are to survive the constraints of physician control. Physician-nurse competition could potentially lead to the demise of the nurse practitioner role. (1982:30)

Among the clinical sites that nurse practitioners are exploring are corporations, schools, public agencies, nursing homes, and other long-term care settings (Aiken, 1981; Ford, 1979; Billingsley and Harper, 1982). Nurse practitioners are also recruiting students from the ranks of nurses in these nontraditional settings because they would be in a good position to demonstrate to their employees how they might benefit their organizations. With nurse practitioners adopting these new and more politically sophisticated strategies in their fight for professional survival, it would be a mistake for pediatricians to underestimate the potential threat that PNPs might present in the future.

A serious glut of primary care pediatricians and increased competition from other health care workers, then, may succeed where the pediatric leadership has failed in making the new morbidity a more prominent feature of pediatric practice. As the size of the child and adolescent population stabilizes and the number of child health care providers, including pediatricians, increases, there will be pressure on primary care pediatricians to pay more attention to the new morbidity as a matter of survival.

At the same time the specialty seems to be considering even more radical changes in its scope of practice to expand the opportunities for primary care pediatricians. Some pediatricians have argued that given the specialty's current interest in teenage sexuality and pregnancy, pelvic examinations, drug abuse, and sports medicine, 21 years of age is an artificial and arbitrary point at which to cut off care to patients. Thompson (1984:807), a former president of the AAP, suggested more than a decade ago that "extending beyond 21 to 25 or 30 years of age may well seem logical in a few years." In its most recent statement on the age limits of pediatrics, the AAP has in fact taken the position that under special circumstances pediatricians should consider providing services for their patients past the age of 21 (AAP, 1988).

Joel Alpert (1990:657), a key proponent for primary care pediatrics, has noted that "pediatric patients have traditionally been age restricted but, continuing the present trend in the future, they will be far less so." He predicts that "tomorrow's pediatrician may well be the family physician for young families. The pediatrician's major responsibility for health care should be providing services for young families with children."

Some pediatricians are reconsidering the proposal that Morse (1937) presented facetiously decades earlier—that pediatricians pursue careers in geriatrics instead of pediatrics. Elizabeth McAnarney (1986:866), chief of the Division of General Pediatrics and Adolescent Medicine at the University of Rochester, has suggested that in light of the growing number of elderly, the undersupply of doctors to care for them, and the oversupply problem that pediatricians are facing, pediatricians should be encouraged to leave pediatrics, train in geriatrics, and subsequently become geriatricians. McAnarney feels that with all the parallels between the young and old, the idea makes sense. Both adolescents and the elderly are undergoing rapid physical and psychological change; for both, identity, independence, and control are key issues; and, like geriatricians, pediatricians are developmentally oriented doctors who relate to "dependent persons, persons who have deficits, and persons who may be limited in their verbal communication." McAnarney believes that a 1 to 2 year educational program would be sufficient to accomplish the transition in careers. Carrying over the comprehensive approach of pediatrics, she adds, the programs would stress the strengths of "successful aging" as well as covering the treatment of illnesses and matters related to death. The "striking" parallels between adolescent medicine and geriatrics have been noted as well by Zack (1981:732).

A move in any of these directions raises questions about whether primary care pediatricians would ultimately retain their identity as pediatricians. If their focus shifts toward young adults and young families, primary care pediatricians may yet merge with family practice. If they take on the problems of the elderly, a less likely but plausible possibility, they may create a new type of primary health care provider with a special expertise in developmental issues. Both scenarios would mean an end to primary care pediatrics as such. Pediatrics would become the kind of consulting specialty that many of the specialty's academic community think it should be.

Whatever the future holds for primary care pediatrics, two things are clear. First, pediatrics is still at a critical juncture in its development and more change is inevitable. Second, however the specialty refashions itself, whatever shape it next takes, and whoever next assumes responsibility for the health care needs of children and adolescents, those responsibilities will include their psychosocial and emotional concerns. The behaviors and misbehaviors of children and young people, for the time being at least, seem firmly entrenched within a medical paradigm.

Chapter 7

Conclusion and Theoretical Considerations

NEW MISSIONS AND TRANSFORMATIONS

The story of the new pediatrics is essentially the story of a profession establishing itself on new turf. In the wake of the dramatic declines in childhood mortality and morbidity, and with the growing emphasis on prevention and well-child care, pediatrics faced a crisis. Primary care pediatricians were willing to do some preventive work. But many felt that in providing preventive services, or even in treating children's minor illnesses, they were not practicing their specialty. They saw prevention and well-child care only as a way to subsidize the "real" work of the specialty—the treatment of serious childhood diseases. From their point of view, pediatrics had exhausted its mission. Most children in North America were safe from the perils of disease. Those who were seriously sick had hospital-based subspecialists to treat them. Prevention did not justify the continued existence of primary care pediatricians. Primary care pediatrics had become, as one practitioner put it, "a specialty that does not exist" (Wineberg, 1959:1008). The specialty needed a new mission.

Pediatrics found that new mission in ministering to the behavioral and psychosocial, rather than simply physical, problems of children and in taking on adolescents as patients. The move to the new pediatrics (or new morbidity in pediatrics) has occurred neither naturally, nor easily. There were in the beginning and there continue to be those who oppose the shift. But the debate about whether pediatricians can or should handle psychosocial problems or the concerns of adolescents has been overshadowed by the more pressing question of whether pediatrics can survive as a primary care specialty. An oversupply of pediatricians and the emergence of other groups of child health care workers ready to provide broad, comprehensive health care to the young have pushed the specialty toward the new pediatrics and are likely to continue to do so.

The problem is not new for pediatricians. The dilemma that has confronted them since the 1950s is not unlike the earlier chapter in the specialty's history when the problems related to the artificial feeding of infants disappeared and pediatricians lost their baby feeding role. The specialty survived then by redefining pediatricians as guardians of child health and moving into prevention. Pediatricians added the supervision of healthy children to their traditional mission of treating sick children and managing difficult feeding problems. While the shift into prevention resolved the question of the specialty's future and continued growth at the time, however, it also set the stage for the crises I have analyzed in this book.

There are parallels between pediatricians and other groups who, facing the elimination or fulfillment of their original goals, need to find new purpose in order to survive. When pharmaceutical companies made the traditional pharmacists' skills of compounding drug products in retail and hospital pharmacies obsolete—producing disenchantment and a crisis of purpose similar to that faced by pediatricians—the profession created the new role of "clinical pharmacist." Clinical pharmacists stress their function as information providers and drug consultants to both physicians and patients (Birenbaum, 1990; Broadhead and Facchinetti, 1985).

Organizational sociologists refer to this phenomenon as "goal succession" (Etzioni, 1964:13–14). A classic study of goal succession is David Sills' (1957) analysis of the Foundation for Infantile Paralysis (FIP). The FIP was established to raise funds to support research into infantile paralysis (poliomyelitis) and to assist victims of the disease. Once Jonas Salk developed the vaccine for polio, the FIP became redundant. Rather than disappearing, however, it changed it name to the March of Dimes and found a new objective in fighting arthritis and birth defects. Other examples of goals succession include the Red Cross, whose initial concerns revolved around wars and other national emergencies, but after World War I became involved in public health (Dulles, 1950), and religious organizations that have added social and community service to their original spiritual mandate.

There are parallels as well between pediatricians and social movements that have transformed themselves. Gerber and Short (1984) document the history of a movement to stem the dangerous and unethical marketing practices of companies supplying infant food formulas to third world countries—the Infant Formula Action Coalition (INFACT). INFACT was formed in 1977 and initiated "a national campaign aimed at changing the practices of American companies and the Swiss giant, Nestle" (Gerber and Short, 1984:12). INFACT led a 7-year boycott of Nestle products and eventually forced the company to alter and restrict its marketing tactics. In the aftermath of its victory, INFACT broadened its objectives. A later mission statement described the coalition as a "peoples' organization building international campaigns to stop abuses of transnational corporations which endanger the health and survival of people all over the world, and particularly threaten third world people by creating enforceable agreements with these corporations" (Gerber and Short, 1984:26).

These professions, organizations, and movements share with pediatricians the experience of having to reinvent themselves to survive. But in doing so, most promote new views of the behaviors and/or conditions they take on as goals. As part of their campaign to fashion a role for clinical pharmacists on health care teams, for example, pharmacists have identified the problem of "drug iatrogenesis"—illnesses caused by errors in the prescription of medications. In similar ways, the March of Dimes, the Red Cross, and groups like INFACT have drawn public attention to a broad range of previously unnoticed health issues. And pediatricians, as I argued in my introduction, have fundamentally altered children's "misbehaviors" and adolescents' "growing pains." Each group, in its efforts to ensure survival, has implicated itself in a process of constructing and promoting a view of the world. It was an interest in pediatricians as claimsmakers and, more specifically, in their participation in the generation and promotion of medical labels for childhood deviance that sparked my interest in the new pediatrics. I want, in the remainder of this chapter, to situate this study in the constructionist literature that frames this study and to discuss the significance of my analysis for the study of social problems and the sociology of professions.

THE CONSTRUCTION OF SOCIAL PROBLEMS

My approach to the new pediatrics has drawn on a perspective in sociology that focuses on how meanings are produced about "undesirable" social conditions, circumstances, or behaviors. This perspective— social constructionism—emerged in the study of social problems, although it can be, and has been, applied to the study of social movements, deviance, and the professions. Rather than looking at "objective conditions" as social problems per se, or as harmful, unjust, dangerous, or inherently undesirable—an approach to the study of social problems that characterized the field till the 1970s—constructionists are interested in how these putative conditions and behaviors come to be seen as social problems (Best, 1989a; Gusfield, 1975, 1981, 1984; Kitsuse, 1980; Schneider, 1985; Schneider and Kitsuse, 1984; Spector and Kitsuse, 1977 [1987]).

The constructionist perspective traces its origins to symbolic interactionism and the writings of George Herbert Mead (1934) and Herbert Blumer (1969). Mead and Blumer argued that the world is not imbued with intrinsic meaning. Social actors give meaning to, or interpret, the objects, situations, and people around them, and then respond to these meanings. They form these meanings in the context of interaction. The meanings are social products, created in and through the defining or interpretive activities of individuals as they interact and try to fit their lines of action to each other. Moreover, these meanings are never fixed. People are constantly adjusting, revising, and modifying the meanings that they attribute to the actions of others. Interaction becomes a constant process of interpreting, negotiating, and renegotiating meanings.

In *Constructing Social Problems*, a book that presents an early statement of constructionism and that has been described as a "watershed in the development of the contemporary sociology of social problems" (Miller and Holstein, 1993:2), Spector and Kitsuse (1977 [1987]) encourage sociologists to abandon the notion that social problems are a kind of condition and proposed instead that social problems are an activity. They defined social problems as "the activities of individuals or groups making grievances and claims with respect to some putative conditions" (1977:75). The task for sociologists, they suggested, was not to evaluate or assess the accuracy of such claims but to account for claimsmaking activity and its results in terms of who gains ownership over certain "social problems" and what policies and institutionalized procedures are established to deal with the putative problem.

The constructionist perspective has generated both a lively theoretical debate and an impressive body of empirical work (see Pawluch, 1996 for a quick overview). The theoretical debate involves the underlying and unstated assumptions that the approach makes, the way it is applied, and the future directions it might take.

The empirical work examines claimsmaking efforts around such issues as prostitution (Jenness, 1993), rape (Rose, 1977), smoking (Troyer, 1989), sexual harassment (Gillespie and Leffler, 1987), wife battery (Tierney, 1982), AIDS (Albert, 1989), rock music (Gray, 1989), drunk driving (Gusfield, 1975; 1981), earthquake risks (Stallings, 1995), and food (Mauer and Sobal, 1995). Many of the case studies show that the claims being made about problematic social conditions are increasingly medical in nature. In other words, there has been a trend toward viewing undesirable conditions, situations, and behaviors as medical problems (Conrad, 1992). A medical vocabulary describes the putative problems and proposed solutions or controls. Indeed, constructionists argue that the medical model dominates the current discourse about social problems. They have documented how this has occurred in a variety of settings including "mental illness" (Conrad and Schneider,

1980a), problem drinking or "alcoholism" (Schneider, 1978), compulsive gambling (Rosecrance, 1985), transsexualism (Billings and Urban, 1982), physician impairment (Morrow, 1982), and cult membership (Robbins and Anthony, 1982).

Constructionists' observations about medicalization are consistent with those of sociologists of medicine who point out that the trend toward medicalization has not been restricted simply to problematic or deviant behaviors but has taken in nonproblematic behaviors as well (Arney and Bergen, 1984). Life itself is becoming medicalized "as medicine wraps itself around more and more categories of behaviors, defining, labeling, diagnosing and treating both physical and mental attributes and actions" (Erchak and Rosenfeld, 1989:79). Zola (1972:487) refers to the trend as "making medicine and the labels 'healthy' and 'ill' relevant to an every increasing part of human existence." Sedgwick (1973:37) has called it "the progressive annexation of nonillness into illness." Ivan Illich (1976), one of the most provocative opponents of medicalization, has accused the medical profession of turning the whole human life span into a series of age-specific disabilities requiring medical supervision. From the unborn and newborn, to the menopausal and old, the entire population is at risk: "Life is turned into a pilgrimage through check-ups and clinics, back to the ward where it started" (1976:87).

For Freidson (1970a) medicalization is a function of the inherent bias in medicine toward the imputation of disease. The medical profession is prone to see illness and the need for treatment more than it is prone to see health and normality. This bias operates both at the interactional level, in doctors' contacts with individual patients, and at the level of generating entirely new categories of disease:

> [The medical profession] is active in seeking out illness. The profession does not only treat the illness laymen take to it, but it also seeks to discover illness of which laymen may not even be aware. One of the greatest ambitions of the physician is to discover and describe a "new" disease" or syndrome and to be immortalized by having his name used to identify the disease. Medicine, then, is oriented to seeking out and finding illness, which is to say that it seeks to create social meaning of illness where that meaning or interpretation was lacking before. (Freidson, 1970a:252)

In their analysis of the medicalization of deviant behaviors, Conrad and Schneider (1980a) argue that disease labels for problem behaviors are only the latest in a progression of paradigmatic shifts in deviance designations. While deviant behaviors have always existed, they point out, the ways in which that deviance has been designated has changed. Prior to the seventeenth century, when a theological world view predominated, deviance tended to be understood as a moral transgression.

With the emergence of the nation-state and the formalization of law, legal or criminal definitions of deviance held sway. The development of modern rationalism and the ascendancy of science have brought with them the inclination to see deviance as a technical, scientific, or medical problem. Deviance designations generally, and medical labels for deviance more specifically, are "the products of a political process, social constructions usually implemented and legitimated by powerful and influential interests and applied to relatively powerless and subordinate groups" (1980a:36). In each case of medicalization, therefore, one needs to consider the definers, the claims they make, the activities in which they engage, and the sociohistorical circumstances surrounding their claimsmaking activities.

CHILDREN, PEDIATRICIANS, AND MEDICALIZATION

Certain groups have been particularly vulnerable to the medical labeling of their behaviors and circumstances. Women are one such group (Bell, 1987; Figert, 1995; McCrea, 1983; Riessman, 1983; Riessman and Nathanson, 1986; Scritchfield, 1989). Children are another. Conrad and Schnieder (1980a) suggest that the relative powerlessness of women and children and their limited ability to resist medicalization have made them prime targets. Several studies examine claimsmaking efforts related specifically to children. While some of these focus on children's problematic behaviors—for example, studies on hyperactivity and learning disabilities (Carrier, 1986; Conrad, 1975; Conrad and Schneider, 1980a; Erchak and Rosenfeld, 1989) and juvenile delinquency (Conrad and Schneider, 1980a)—others have examined issues that are, in other ways, child-related, including child abuse (Johnson, 1989; Parton, 1979; Pfohl, 1977), missing children (Best, 1987, 1989b, 1990), abducted children (Gentry, 1988), sudden infant death syndrome (Johnson and Hufbauer, 1982), child custody and child support laws (Coltrane and Hickman, 1992), and accidental poisoning (Broadhead, 1986). Margolin (1994) traces the creation of the "gifted child" concept and shows how the concept has affected the way *all* children are seen. As Margolin (1994:105) points out, "it is impossible to make the gifted's "superiority" happen or appear without a conceptualization of a comparison group."

Many of these studies touch on the role played by the medical profession and its tacit approval of, if not active involvement in, the campaigns that turned these issues into public concerns. Conrad (1975, 1976), in his analysis of hyperactivity, points out that once certain forms of childhood deviance were labeled as "hyperkinesis" or "hyperactivity," the medical profession assumed the responsibility for managing and controlling it and that, although it may not have sought this role, "its members have been, in general, disturbingly unconcerned and unquestioning in their acceptance of it" (Conrad, 1975:52).

Some studies single out pediatricians as key players. Broadhead (1986:426) argues that pediatricians were the first to draw attention to poisoning as "an alarming danger to children" and were at the forefront of the poison control movement. In fact, the first poison control center, established in 1953, was organized in Chicago under the sponsorship of the Illinois chapter of the American Academy of Pediatrics. Broadhead cites a paper in the *Journal of the American Medical Association* reviewing the development of poison control over 5 years after the first center was established. The paper noted: "Probably the most noteworthy of these developments is the realization by the medical profession, especially by pediatricians, that poison accidents constitute a major health problem" (Cann and Verhulst, in Broadhead, 1986:426).

Pfohl's (1977) analysis of the "discovery" of child abuse concentrates on the central role played by pediatric radiologists. But Pfohl notes that pediatric radiologists were supported in their campaign to bring the child abuse problem to light by pediatricians and psychiatrists. Both specialties, he insists, enjoyed marginal status within medical ranks and felt that a link with the "deadly forces of abuse" could enlarge the risky part of their mission and thereby reduce their marginality.

But none of the studies examines the forces that propelled pediatricians to involve themselves in the medicalization of so many childhood issues or at the critical stake that the specialty had in the redefinition of behaviors that once fell beyond the medical purview. This study shows that pediatricians' involvement in the seemingly relentless medicalization of children's lives was linked to the crises that the specialty faced over the past half century and their efforts to adapt to the changing circumstances around them. The new pediatrics was rooted not in any naturally expansionary, "carnivorous" (Abbott, 1988:87) or imperialistic tendencies of the medical profession to extend its privileges and prerogatives—a conclusion that some analysts come to about medicalization (Strong, 1979)—but in the concerns of a primary care specialty struggling to survive. An understanding of the dilemmas that pediatricians faced and the professional concerns that have preoccupied them since the 1950s is critical to understanding their involvement in the medicalization of children's deviant behaviors and other problems in their lives.

PROFESSIONS AS CLAIMSMAKERS

In theoretical terms, the new pediatrics provides an opportunity to reflect more generally on professions as claimsmakers—the circumstances under which a profession undertakes claimsmaking activity, the shape that professional claimsmaking takes, and the difficulties that medical claimsmaking (or medicalization), as a strategy for resolving professional problems, can generate for a profession.

The new pediatrics underscores first, the extent to which claimsmaking around social problems can become enmeshed with professional concerns, and, therefore, points out the need to look at claimsmaking in the context of professional development. In this regard, the sociology of professions has insights to offer. The sociological study of professions was once characterized by a preoccupation with how professions are different from other occupations. Endless lists of distinguishing characteristics were produced with little agreement, in the end, about what traits the lists should include (Millerson, 1964) and little discussion of how such lists advanced an understanding of the professions or their role in society. Over the past several decades, however, sociologists have found a different way to think about professions. Rooted in interactionist critiques of the "trait" approach (Ritzer and Walczak, 1986) offered by such sociologists as Everett Hughes (1951, 1961, 1971), Howard Becker (1962), and Julius Roth (1974)—and influenced by many of the same ideas that gave rise to the constructionist approach to social problems—the more recent view of professions shifts the focus away from the identification of professional traits. Instead, the concern is to explain how professions emerge, develop, and change, and how—as a part of that process—they may seek the label "professional," professional status, and its incumbent rewards.

Rue Bucher, who along with Anselm Strauss first proposed this image of "professions in process" (Bucher, 1962; Bucher and Strauss, 1961:325), has developed a natural history model of professional development (Bucher, 1980; 1988). Professions, she suggests, organize, consolidate, and then often transform as they face threats to their existence and look for ways to rejuvenate themselves. At each stage in their development there are unique problems to overcome and issues to resolve. Emerging groups need to worry about developing a clear identity and ideology to rationalize their work, establishing their legitimacy, attracting recruits, and building training programs. Consolidating groups must deal with the problems that come along with increased organizational complexity. Transforming professions need to renegotiate their relationships with client groups, with the formal organizations within which they work and with other occupations. The activities of a transforming profession can resemble those of emerging professions.

Andrew Abbott (1988) has also produced concepts and a theoretical framework that can be useful in studying professions as claimsmakers. Abbott argues that professions exist within a system and that their histories are inevitably interdependent. Within this system, jurisdictional boundaries are in constant dispute. "It is the history of jurisdictional disputes," he (1988:2) insists, "that is the real, the determining history of the professions."

It is against this backdrop of ongoing professional development and perpetual jurisdictional disputes that professional claimsmaking occurs and needs to be understood. The new pediatrics was essentially a revitalization formula for a profession threatened by challenges of various sorts to its jurisdictional boundaries. The broadening of the pediatric mandate was initially a way for pediatricians to salvage a meaningful role for those in primary care at a time when practitioners were questioning their usefulness, and later, a way to justify the contributions of primary care pediatrics in an increasingly competitive child health care market. Any account of medicalization as it has affected the lives of children would be incomplete without some comprehension of these fundamental dilemmas and the factors that drove pediatricians' claims making around children.

Second, the new pediatrics raises questions about the forms that professional claimsmaking can take. Conrad and Schneider (1980a:266–271) talk about the discovery of new medical diseases and the creation of medical diagnoses as claimsmaking. Another, more obvious, form that claimsmaking takes is social or political activism in relation to issues that a profession feels strongly about and that it often claims it is uniquely equipped to solve. Pediatricians, individually and collectively, have engaged in both types of claimsmaking. They have been among the "discoverers" of specific new behavioral conditions in children and have participated in the political campaigns that have brought such issues as child abuse, seat belt use, and accidental poisoning to light as social problems. [There are parallels here to Aronson's (1982, 1984) discussions of claimsmaking among scientists.]

But the incorporation of so many childhood and adolescent difficulties within a medical frame of reference was more subtly the consequence of a redrawing of the boundaries of pediatric practice. In changing and expanding their definition of their political task, pediatricians cleared the way for the production of specific disease labels and for political activism on the part of pediatricians as well as others. This suggests that forms that professional claimsmaking can take, and how various forms relate to each other, need to be more clearly specified. We need a better understanding not only of why professions become involved in the social problems process, but in what ways they do so.

Finally, this analysis of the new pediatrics points out that in looking at professional claimsmaking, we need to remember that professions are not monolithic, bound by a common purpose and common interests, speaking in one voice and acting always in concert. Professions are more accurately described as loose groupings of workers representing a plurality of interests and a diversity of views. Bucher and Strauss (1961) call these groupings "segments." They point out that these segments differ from each other in significant ways and that they can, and often do, come into conflict with each other over everything from the profession's fundamental mission and the clients it should be serving, to the methods and techniques the profession should be using. Abbott's (1988:117–142) work on the professions also highlights the internal differentiation that can characterize professions and the disturbances that these divisions can create for the profession.

The division in pediatrics between primary care generalists and pediatric subspecialists, practitioners, and academics, the organizational leaders of the profession and its rank and file are all key to the development of the new pediatrics. These same divisions explain the tensions that the new pediatrics has generated and the uneven enthusiasm within the specialty for the idea of a broader scope of practice. While for some, the new pediatrics offers the specialty its best hope for survival as a primary care specialty, for others it threatens to diminish pediatrics' status and legitimacy as an academic discipline within medicine. This study shows that medicalization, as a strategy for professional rejuvenation, can create as many difficulties for a profession as it solves if it interferes with the separate interests of its constituent segments. And in analyzing professional claimmaking, to overlook the segments that make up a profession and the relationship of these segments to each other would be to miss much of the dynamic that may be fueling or impeding claimsmaking efforts.

Appendix

This appendix has several purposes. On the simplest level, I want to describe how I traced the development of the new pediatrics—the steps I took, the research techniques I used, and the data I gathered. In the process of researching and writing the book, however, I learned not just about pediatricians, but about studying professions as claimsmakers. A second purpose, then, is to suggest strategies for those interested in undertaking similar work—to identify the places one might look for insights into the professional concerns that often drive professional claimsmaking and the internal debates that typically accompany such claimsmaking. Last, I address briefly some of the methodological and conceptual problems that this, or any constructionist study, poses in relation to how to think about data, and situate my work in this book in the context of current debates about the use of the constructionist perspective.

SOURCES OF DATA

The data for this analysis came from a variety of sources, the most central of which was pediatrics' own literature—its journals, monographs, textbooks, conference proceedings, organizational policy statements and promotional literature, surveys, newsletters, committee reports, training manuals, and other educational materials, and internal histories, biographies, and autobiographies, that is, those written by pediatricians principally for their pediatric colleagues. The journals were particularly important. I systematically examined several journals including *Pediatrics*, the official journal of the American Academy of Pediatrics, the *Journal of Pediatrics*, and the *American Journal of the Diseases of Children* from their first to their most current issues, and for the specialty's early history, the *Archives of Pediatrics*, the *Transactions of the American Pediatric Society*, and the *Transactions of the Section on the Diseases of Children*. I paid special attention to editorials, letters to the editor, commentaries, debates, presidential addresses, addresses by recipients of major awards, and the news and announcement sections of the journals. I also consulted the professional literature of groups such as family practitioners and pediatric nurse practitioners to get a sense for the developments on those field that were pertinent to pediatrics.

I supplemented these materials with a variety of other data. I looked at both historical and current census data describing general patterns in infancy, child and maternal mortality rates, life expectancy, morbidity, and birth rates. To explain the demographic trends and to place developments in pediatrics in their larger sociohistorical context, I turned to a vast body of historical and sociological work on such topics as the public health movement, the child and maternal welfare movement, the emergence of medical specialties, the development of organized medicine, and the current health care system.

Sydney Halpern's (1982, 1988, 1990) sociological analyses of American pediatrics deserve special mention. In a book titled *American Pediatrics: The Social Dynamics of Professionalism, 1880–1980* (1988), Halpern looks mostly at pediatrics' early years. She uses pediatrics to examine broader questions of professional evolution and change. Her book stresses the structural conditions that generate new work patterns within professions over the claimsmaking activities of professional segments. Nevertheless, her account of pediatrics' history was useful as I mapped out the developments that serve as a backdrop for the emergence of the new pediatrics. A later paper (Halpern, 1990) focuses specifically on the last four decades in pediatrics and provides a nice discussion of how the emphasis on behavioral and psychosocial problems in pediatrics may mean competition between social scientists and pediatricians for research support.

I interviewed several retired pediatricians who entered their specialty's ranks during the 1930s and 1940s, and whose careers spanned the periods of significant change in the specialty's history. As well, I interviewed general pediatricians in private, primary care practices, pediatricians who specialize in the treatment of behavioral and learning problems, residents in pediatrics, one of whom was in the process of transferring from pediatrics to child psychiatry, interns who were considering pediatrics as an area of specialty practice, a psychologist who works with behaviorally disturbed children in a pediatric hospital, general and family practitioners, and pediatric nurse practitioners. There were about 30 formal interviews. I have not included countless, more casual conversations with pediatricians, other health care workers, and parents. I have had many opportunities over the years it has taken to do this study to present my work to both medical and nonmedical audiences. These presentations invariably elicited observations, reactions, opinions, and anecdotal experiences that were illuminating. For the most part, they confirmed trends and patterns that I had already detected in the literature. However, in some cases, they sensitized me to issues that I had overlooked or the significance of which I had missed.

To get a clearer sense of what the practice of pediatrics actually entails, I spent time as a participant observer in a variety of settings: private pediatric practices, various wards and clinics of a children's hospital, most notably a Learning Disorder Clinic and a Behavioral Pediatrics Clinic, several family medicine clinics in general hospitals, and the meetings of a pediatric research team comprised of pediatric specialists and subspecialists, epidemiologists, and social scientists. I also spent 2 days with a general pediatrician practicing in a relatively isolated community. As one of only two pediatricians in the community, she functioned primarily as a referral specialist, and dealt with problems that, in most urban settings, would have fallen under the purview of a subspecialist. Like the interviews, the data from these observations did not find their way directly into the book. But they were useful indirectly in rounding out my understanding of the key issues in pediatrics today. They also showed me how the decisions made at an official or organization level have affected the practice of pediatrics.

THE PROFESSIONAL LITERATURE: "VOICES IN THE LIBRARY"

I argued in my conclusion that studying professional claimsmaking amounts inevitably to looking at professional development. And the discussion about my data sources makes obvious the extent to which I relied on pediatrics' own literature. I want, here, to make a more explicit case for the value of the professional literature as a source of information about the professions. Sociologists who study professions, while not oblivious to the professional literature, have tended until recently to use this literature in limited ways—to supplement or provide background information for interviews and direct observation, to cover the historical aspects of a profession's development, or as a "pathway" (Habenstein, 1970) to other types of data. Habenstein (1970), for example, in discussing ways to study the professions, deals almost exclusively with strategies for making and deepening contacts with its members. He directs the attention of investigators to journals in the field, but only as a way of identifying possible contacts. Journal editors, he points out, should be sought out because they are usually "in the know" and may themselves be involved in movements within the profession that a sociologist might want to explore. The "lowly letter to the editor" (Habenstein, 1970:108) is a good place to discover the rank and file zealots. If they were willing to write a letter to the editor, he speculates, they would probably be willing to talk to a sociologist. Why letters to the editor are "lowly" and why they cannot stand on their own, as data on rank and file positions within the profession, are not clear.

This relative neglect of the professional literature reflects a more general aversion within sociology to documentary data. Glaser and Strauss (1967), who treat written documents as a way of generating "grounded" theory in sociology, offer a range of explanations for the aversion. They suggest that it might have to do with (1) the traditional concern, at least in American sociology, to clearly separate the social sciences from the interests and methods of history, which many regard as a more humanistic field; (2) sociologists' desire to see the concrete situations and individuals they are studying; and (3) sociologists' distrust of their competence in discovering and working with documentary materials. "The well-trained sociologist," they write (1967:163), "may brave the rigors of the field or confront the most recalcitrant interviewees, but quail before the library." They go on to encourage a more serious consideration of these materials:

> When someone stands in the library stacks, he is, metaphorically, surrounded by voices begging to be heard. Every book, every magazine article represents at least one person who is equivalent to the anthropologist's informant, or the sociologist's interviewee. In those publications, people converse, announce positions, argue with a range of eloquence, and describe events or scenes in ways entirely comparable to what is seen and heard during field work. The researcher needs only to discover the *voices in the library* to release them for his analytic use. (1967:163; emphasis added)

I discovered these *voices in the library* serendipitously. I started my research, as many sociologists do, intending to use the library only to gather the information I needed to ensure a productive foray into "the field." As my search continued, however, I gradually realized that "the field," as it were, lay in the various documents I was uncovering, especially the literature generated by and for pediatricians.

I found information on virtually every aspect of pediatrics' development. For every phase of the specialty's history, from its formative years as an organized specialty to the present, I found descriptions of key turning points and milestones, discussions of the issues that preoccupied its practitioners, debates about the course that the specialty should be following, and surveys relating to both practice patterns and pediatricians' views on a broad range of subjects. I found the clearest expressions, for example, of pediatricians' claims about the unmet, nonphysical health care needs of children and teenagers, the seriousness of those needs, and their own capacity as doctors to address them.

As well, I found information on trends outside pediatrics—i.e., government policies and demographic shifts in the population of children— that pediatricians felt were bound to affect their work. Professional groups, I discovered, can be extremely sensitive to changes in their environment. They are quick to pick up on such trends, and thorough in exploring their potential implications. Beyond documenting profession-al claimsmaking, then, these materials allow one to get a glimpse of the context for professions' claimsmaking—the circumstances under which these activities are undertaken, how the group coordinates its claims making activities with its professional interests, the in-house debates, behind-the-scenes maneuvering and wrangling involved in formulating professional strategies, and the discussions about how to present a co-herent and unified position to outside audiences.

Pediatricians' books, reports, and journals were filled with discus-sions about the challenges that pediatricians saw themselves facing, the options they considered, and the directions that various segments of the profession felt the specialty ought to follow. The "dissatisfied pediatrician syndrome" was a phenomenon that revealed itself first in the form of letters to the editors of pediatric journals, and was then confirmed by surveys conducted and published by those same jour-nals. The image that pediatricians hoped to promote as the new pedi-atrics evolved, and the rhetoric they used to justify their new roles and interests, were also reflected in their own literature. The contents of the new pediatrics took shape in the specialty's training manuals and educational materials.

Presidential addresses were particularly revealing, as their titles alone suggest—"Whither Pediatrics?" (Low, 1977), "Pediatrics at the Delta" (Holt, 1961), "Pediatrics: A Perspective on the Present and Future of a Proud Profession" (Olmsted, 1978), "Pediatric Education at the Cross-roads" (Levine, 1960), "American Pediatrics—A Retrospect and Fore-cast" (Holt, 1923), and "Pediatrics in the Space Age" (Cole, 1959). Many offered a thoughtful, considered, and reflexive stock-taking of the spe-cialty, its problems, and its prospects.

Perhaps such stock-taking has to do with what presidential addresses are supposed to be about. In any organization the position of president is honorific and prestigious. It is a symbol of its incumbent's status as a respected and admired leader in the field. The membership of the orga-nization expects from its presidents the kind of statement that they, by virtue of their experience, authority, perspective, and, sometimes, wis-dom, are uniquely qualified to make. Presidents are usually painfully aware of these expectations and from the moment of their election begin to collect their thoughts about the kind of speech they might want to deliver. They usually strive for a momentous statement, one befitting a president, and one that will make an impact. As Erving Goffman (1983:1) wrote, reflecting on his own 1982 address to the American So-ciological Association—an address he was unable to actually deliver due to illness, but one that was printed in the association's journal—: "in theory, a presidential address, whatever its character, must have significance for the profession, even if only a sad one."

Or perhaps such addresses are a sign of crisis within a profession. When the profession is going through relatively stable periods in its development, presidents have the luxury of basking in its past glories and accomplishments, paying tribute to past presidents, ruminating on technical discoveries or research frontiers, or focusing on such matters as the organization's finances and activities during their tenure as president. There have been presidential addresses from pediatricians that have fallen into each of these categories. But when the profession is experiencing difficulties and an uncertain future, there is pressure for its leaders to deal with the crisis at hand. These are the moments in its history when members of a professional organization look to their leaders for direction and guidance. They do not want to hear empty platitudes about the profession's greatness, but frank and realistic analyses of its problems. They want to be reassured that their leaders are sensitive to these problems and have some vision to guide the profession through turbulent times.

In either case, when presidential addresses take the form of stock-taking, they are a valuable resource for those who study professions. They allow analysts to take the pulse of the profession, and to get an idea of how far the profession feels it has come and where it feels it is going. The professions themselves seem to recognize the significance of these addresses as a record of their development. Pediatricians, for example, have, from time to time, published their presidential addresses in the form of collections. On the twenty-fifth anniversary of the AAP, Beaven (1955) brought together, in one volume, the addresses of the organization's first 25 presidents. In their history of the APS, Faber and McIntosh (1966) devote a chapter to tracing the main themes of its presidential addresses over the period 1889–1964. Such collections make it relatively easy to map out the course that a specialty or profession has followed over the years.

The more one learns about the professional literature, the more systematic one can be in exploring it. Many of my initial finds were what Glaser and Strauss (1967:164) call "lucky accidents." Besides using subject catalogues and computerized searches to locate relevant data, I spent hours in the library looking at titles that looked promising or going through pediatric journals. I always stumbled across material I could use. As I became more familiar with the literature, however, I developed a better sense of where to look for the material I needed. I learned, for example, that certain journals are the main repository for the committee reports and official policy statements of professional organizations; that the preface of textbooks and monographs, as well as the inaugural issue of new, specialized journals can yield useful information about how professions would describe the "state of the art" within their fields; that professional organizations often commemorate an anniversary by publishing a festschrift, a history of the organization, collections of biographies, or a series of essays on historical or contemporary issues in the profession—all of which can be informative; that certain individuals can be counted on to argue a particular point of view consistently over the years and that by tracing their contributions, and the reactions to them, one can get a sense of the relative strength of their position within the profession; and, as I have pointed out, that presidential addresses can be like windows on a profession, providing a clear view of current preoccupations and concerns.

The "voices in the library," in the form of the professional literature, are a particularly valuable resource for constructionists, who emphasize the actors' (professions') perspective. They provide data that would be difficult, if not impossible, to obtain in any other way. Doctors have been notoriously ambivalent, if not outrightly unenthusiastic, about sociologists and their research. They are not like other groups flattered by the attention of scholars, welcoming a sociologist's interest, and perhaps anxious for the credibility that they feel such attention might lend to their causes. As Rosengren (1980:87) puts it, while the mere uttering of the words "professor" or "sociologist" is enough to "open doors and mouths" among other groups, doctors are less likely to be impressed. Rosengren attributes doctors' reticence to the public image of sociologists as scholars with "soft" methodologies and radical politics. "At the very least," he argues (1980:89), "the approaching sociologist is easily regarded either as an "outsider" who carries some generalized kind of "threat" or as a relatively benign bungler who has little to offer."

A review of Sydney Halpern's (1988) history of pediatrics, written by a doctor and published in *The New England Journal of Medicine* (Hubbell, 1989), provides support for Rosen's contention. Dr. John P. Hubbell describes Halpern as "an obviously competent sociologist who appears to have a rather jaundiced view of pediatrics, and probably of the entire medical profession." The review ends sarcastically: "Although I must respect the author's right to her point of view, I feel that it is overwhelmingly one-sided. I wonder why?" (Hubbell, 1989:1358).

Whatever its source, doctors' aversion to outside scrutiny has been heightened in recent years with the increased criticism of the medical profession. Doctors have become "familiar whipping boys," Haug (1973:204) points out, for a variety of disaffected groups. There is a growing sense of beleaguerment within the profession that has made doctors even more wary of outsiders' questions. This poses obvious problems for anyone interested in studying the profession. The problems are particularly acute for those, like constructionists, who question how the profession might be involved in the redefinition and medicalization of people's lives. Though the term medicalization does not necessarily imply a challenge to medicial definitions or medical authority over particular conditions, the intentions of those who study medicalization are often interpreted as unfriendly (Strong, 1979).

However, while the medical profession may have become more guarded and sensitive to the kind of public image that it projects, it leaves a richly telling and stunningly candid account of its affairs in the public record. Doctors may be loathe to talk to inquiring sociologists, but in their journals and other published documents they talk openly and freely to each other, and these documents are readily available to the sociologist. The experience of reading the professional literature is just as Glaser and Strauss (1967) describe it—standing like an invisible observer among members of the profession as they debate, consider, reflect on, and make decisions about who they are and where they are going. Furthermore, the data derived from the professional literature is what Webb et al. (1966) would call "unobtrusive." Sociologists get a direct rendering of the profession's view of things, not a sanitized version prepared for public consumption.

Why would the medical profession, so careful about its public image in some ways, reveal itself so openly in its own literature? One explanation, of course, is that the professions do not conceive of their published documents as part of the public record. They assume that their journals and most of the documentary material they generate will circulate primarily among members of the profession. The more compelling explanation is that beyond the earliest stages of its development, a profession has no choice but to use its publications as a forum for discussing its affairs. Once a professional organization is in place, it invariably begins to generate records in the form of minutes, conference proceedings, policy statements, newsletters, annual reports, and journals. The larger the group, the more dependent it is on these documents as a channel of communication among its members. But in making their views and opinions known, and in relaying relevant information to each other through their literature, professionals make this information available to a much larger audience. To paraphrase Glaser and Strauss (1967) again, sociologists need only to avail themselves of these materials to unleash their possibilities as a source of data about professional claimsmaking.

LARGER METHODOLOGICAL ISSUES AND DEBATES

The Socially Constructed Nature of Data

As I have pointed out elsewhere, my study of the new pediatrics falls within a tradition that takes as its fundamental premise that reality is socially constructed. The premise applies not only to the claims that actors make about reality, but to the evidence that they present in support of their claims. This evidence often takes the form of census data, medical statistics, or the results of objective, scientific, or historical studies. The conventional view of such "evidence" or "data" is that they reflect underlying objective trends and realities. While there may be disputes about the accuracy of a particular set of numbers or the findings or conclusions of particular studies, the notion that reality can be captured numerically or through objective research is generally accepted. Evidence, in its various forms, then, is traditionally understood as more or less accurate representations of what is happening in the real world.

Constructionism provides an alternative point of view. From a constructionist perspective, statistics and other "objective" data are part of the claimsmaking process. Social actors may privilege certain claims as "fact," "truth," "scientific findings," or "objective knowledge." But for constructionists they are claims and, therefore, subject to the same scrutiny as other claims. Their value lies not in what they tell us about reality, but in what they tell us about those who produce and use them. Rather than accepting data uncritically as a more or accurate reflection of reality, constructionism suggests that these data should be turned into objects of analysis in their own right.

What implications does this have for the data used in this study—the rates, statistics, and numbers describing levels of birth and fertility, infant, child, and maternal mortality, morbidity, availability of child health care providers, children in various age ranges, the extent of the "dissatisfied pediatrician" problem, the children and teens experiencing psychosocial difficulties etc. or the documentation of assorted historical, demographic, and sociological trends that figure so prominently in the development of the new pediatrics?

Constructionism offers another way to think about these data. From a constructionist perspective one can view them not as indicators of the conditions that pediatricians actually faced, but as constructions that pediatricians *used* in various ways—to ascertain patterns and trends in their environment that they felt were likely to exert an impact on their profession, to assess the nature and degree of their impact, to challenge the claims of others when they felt those claims were contestable and to buttress the claims that they themselves were making.

For example, mortality and morbidity rates, once produced and available for pediatricians and others to use, became part of the symbolic world within which they function. They are part of the "reality" against which pediatricians felt they were reacting and to which they saw themselves responding. The accuracy of these rates, their relationship to reality—even if it could be determined, and questions about whether pediatricians were warranted in their interpretation of these numbers are all irrelevant. The point is that pediatricians accepted these rates unquestioningly as indicators of the changes occurring around them and used them to identify, track, assess, and interpret their environment. Their interpretations, in turn, provide a context or interpretive framework for understanding their actions.

In cases where pediatricians challenged the data of others—when they charged, for example, that the methodology of surveys predicting a glut of pediatricians had a built-in bias against their specialty—the issue is not whether pediatricians were "right" or "wrong," but how they used their interpretations of "good science" to undermine the assertions of others. And when pediatricians produced data of their own, as they did in documenting the prevalence of the behavioral problems that they saw as constituting "the new morbidity," their efforts can be viewed not as an attempt to arrive at an objective measure of these problems, but as part of their strategy to get behavioral problems recognized as medical and pediatric problems.

Beyond offering a different perspective on claims that take the form of data, however, constructionism raises broader questions about such data. Constructionism encourages us to ask how data of various types are produced, by whom, under what circumstances, to what purpose, and with what consequences. When are data more likely to be accepted matter-of-factly as "true?" When are they more likely to be contested? Are there features related to the producers of, or audiences for, data that contribute to their credibility (Ibarra and Kitsuse, 1993)?" There is some work in the constructionist literature that touches directly on such questions. We have some understanding of how official crime statistics are generated (Kitsuse and Cicourel, 1963; Pfohl, 1994:360–364), how documents like the DSM manual are created (Kirk and Kutchins, 1992), how specific conditions, like posttraumatic stress disorder (Scott, 1990), get included in such manuals, and how other behaviors, like homosexuality (Spector, 1977; Spector and Kitsuse, 1977 [1988]), get dropped. We know too how certain medical diagnoses, such as premenstrual syndrome (Figert, 1995) and hyperkinesis (Conrad, 1975; 1976), are created and become available to be counted and treated. For other types of data, such analyses have yet to be done.

Not knowing, in specific terms, how a particular set of numbers or documents came into existence—how they were produced—need not stop us from looking at how they are being used by claimsmakers, so long as we recognize and treat them as the products of claimsmaking activity. Moreover, from a practical point of view, analyses cannot be continuously side-tracked into studying how "facts" that claimsmakers use are created and acquire their facticity. Not all stories can be about "data" production. But the more we understand about how data are constructed, the more careful we can be in treating them as the products of claimsmaking activity and the less likely we are to fall into the trap of thinking about these data as reflections of what is "really going on in the world."

Assumptions about Reality

Of course, the trickier issue raised by constructionism for anyone who uses the perspective is not how claimsmakers use data, but how we, as analysts, do. Is there not a fundamental inconsistency in insisting that the claims made, and data used, by the claimsmakers we study are socially constructed, while we blindly use data ourselves, as a resource and as if these data were indisputable, to study claimsmaking activities? The issue here is one of ontological gerrymandering.

Ontological gerrymandering is a term that Steve Woolgar and I (Woolgar and Pawluch, 1985a,b) used to describe the boundary work that constructionists do in structuring their empirical accounts of claimsmaking processes. We argued that constructionists treat the claims of social actors about the nature of reality as social constructions that need to be explained, but that in providing explanations for these constructions they themselves make assumptions about reality that they count on readers to accept in unchallenging ways. In other words, constructionist accounts highlight and raise questions about the claimsmaking of others, while bracketing or backgrounding the assumptions on which the analysis is based. Ontological gerrymandering is the rhetorical strategy that constructionists use to separate the problematic truth status of those constructions they want to explain from those they want left unexamined.

Consider this book. Ontological gerrymandering is used to problematize the changing conceptions of childhood deviance while assuming the constancy of the childhood behaviors in question. The occurrence of such behaviors and their "deviant" character are taken for granted, while definitions of these behaviors as misbehaviors or medical problems are held up for analysis. I look critically at how pediatricians used "data" to construct interpretations about threats to their survival, yet I used some of the same data uncritically myself to provide a context and explanation for pediatricians' activities. The data matching numbers of children to the numbers of available health care providers are part of the mediated or constructed "reality" within which, I argued, pediatricians find themselves functioning, but at the same time they are the data I use to speculate on the future course of the new pediatrics. In places, the analysis even suggests that pediatricians were either "right" or "wrong" in their assessment of the trends around them. They were "right" in their conclusions about the disaffection among primary care pediatricians through the 1950s, which "surveys showed" was widespread, but "wrong" to take credit for the declines in childhood mortality, which "historical analyses reveal" had more to do with the adoption of public health measures. Determinations of "right" and "wrong" hinge not only on the assumption that reality (the "truth" of the matter) is knowable, but on a particular and fixed construction of that reality. In each case, the ontological boundaries are drawn so as to bring pediatricians' claims making into relief, while minimizing the possibility that my own claims making will be called into question. The relativism that I invoke is selective—it applies to the constructions of others but not to my own.

There has been an intense debate within constructionism about whether this kind of boundary work is avoidable—whether it is possible, or even desirable to study the social world without making assumptions about reality (Best, 1995; Gusfield, 1985; Hazelrigg, 1985; Holstein and Miller, 1993; Miller and Holstein, 1993; Pfohl, 1985; Schneider, 1985b; Troyer, 1992). Not all constructionists are necessarily striving for an assumption-free analysis. For some, the logical and conceptual inconsistencies in constructionists' use of relativism do not detract from the value of the perspective in reorienting our attention from the traditional concerns of sociology with objective realities to the processes by which people, in their interactions with each other, construct meanings (Gusfield, 1985; Rafter, 1992). In other words, we should focus on the upside of constructionism—on the fascinating new questions that immediately present themselves from a constructionist perspective—instead of becoming preoccupied with the downside of the approach.

Among those for whom consistent theory remains a goal, there appears to be a growing consensus that a complete relativism may not be possible—that an assumption-free analysis is unattainable and that explanations for anything cannot be provided without taking some aspect of reality for granted. Some "slippage" into objectivism and some "lapse into relativism" appear inevitable (Best, 1995:343; Sarbin and Kitsuse, 1994:14). For Best (1995), the "slippage" is a matter of the degree. He puts it in terms of how far one "steps back" from objectivism and how far one goes in assuming less and calling still more into question. Best's characterization suggests a scale of theoretical purity that seems itself premised in an objectivist stance: the fewer assumptions we make, the closer we get to the "true" nature of social reality.

Perhaps it is safer to talk not about making more or fewer assumptions, but about the *different* sets of assumptions that constructionists can and do make in getting on with the practical task of explaining. And perhaps it is more productive, as Woolgar and I suggested in our original critique of constructionism, to think of ontological gerrymandering not as signs of slippage and logical inconsistencies (Best, 1995:341) or "flawed theory" (Ibarra and Kitsuse, 1993:29), but as practical accomplishments on the part of those who use the approach. While the theoretical debates about what constructionism is, and can be, continue, constructionists routinely use the perspective to research a broad range of issues and empirical questions. This book is an example. Ontological questions that are, in principle, irresolvable, are managed somehow as decisions are made—more or less carefully and more or less reflexively—about how to get on with the task at hand—examining and explaining claimsmaking processes.

How these decisions are made and with what consequences for the questions that we, as social scientists, pose for ourselves and the kinds of answers we provide are, like questions about the production of data, key to understanding how we construct reality and create meaning. But they are questions with which constructionist have barely begun to grapple. In this sense, the consensus that a "strict," assumption-free constructionism seems unlikely is an occasion for celebration, not despondency. Instead of pursuing the elusive search for perfect theory, we may finally begin to give these questions the attention they deserve.

References

Abbott, Andrew. 1988. *The System of Professions: An Essay on the Division of Expert Labor.* Chicago: University of Chicago Press.

Aiken, Linda H. 1981. Nursing Priorities for the 1980s: Hospitals and Nursing Homes. *American Journal of Nursing* 81(2):324–330.

Albert, Edward. 1989. AIDS and the Press: The Creation and Transformation of a Social Problem. Pp. 39–54 in *Images of Issues: Typifying Contemporary Social Problems,* edited by Joel Best. New York: Aldine de Gruyter.

Aldrich, C. Anderson. 1934. The Composition of Private Pediatric Practice. *American Journal of Diseases of Children* 47(5):1051–1064.

Aldrich, Robert A., and Richard H. Spitz. 1960. Survey of Pediatric Practice in the United States, 1959. Pp. 57–74 in *Careers in Pediatrics,* edited by Richard H. Spitz. Report of the Thirty-sixth Ross Conference on Pediatric Research. Columbus, Ohio: Ross Laboratories.

Alpert, Joel J. 1990. Primary Care: The Future of Pediatric Education. *Pediatrics* 86(5):653–659.

———. 1991. The Future of Primary Care—In Reply. *Pediatrics* 88(1):187–188.

———. 1995. The Ambulatory Pediatric Association. *Pediatrics* 95(3):422–426.

AMA Council on Long Range Planning and Development in Cooperation with the American Academy of Pediatrics. 1987. The Future of Pediatrics: Implications of the Changing Environment of Medicine. *Journal of the AMA* 258(2):240–245.

Ambuel, J. Philip. 1959. Letter to the Editor. *Pediatrics* 23(5):1008–1010.

American Academy of Pediatrics. 1938. Proceedings of the Eighth Annual Meeting. *Journal of Pediatrics* 3(1):127.

———. 1950. Child Health Services and Pediatric Education. Report of the Committee for the Study of Child Health Services. *Pediatrics* 6(3): 509–556.

———. 1967. *Standards of Child Health Care.* Report of the Council on Pediatric Practice. Evanston, Illinois: American Academy of Pediatrics.

———. 1972. *Standards of Child Health Care.* Second Edition. Report of the Committee on Standards of Child Health Care, Evanston, Illinois: American Academy of Pediatrics.

———. 1975. *Pediatric Nurse Associates Practitioners' Scope of Practice.* A Statement by the Committee on Pediatric Manpower. Evanston, Illinois: American Academy of Pediatrics.

———. 1977. *Standards of Child Health Care.* Third Edition. Report of the Committee on Standards of Child Health Care. Evanston, Illinois: American Academy of Pediatrics.

———. 1980. *Demographic and Socioeconomic Fact Book on Child Health Care: A*

Survey of Trends in the United States. Evanston, Illinois: American Academy of Pediatrics.

――――. 1981a. Critique of the Final Report of the Graduate Medical Education National Advisory Committee. *Pediatrics* 67(5):585–596.

――――. 1981b. *American Academy of Pediatrics News and Comments* 32(12):3.

――――. 1982. Pediatrics and the Psychosocial Aspects of Child and Family Health. *Pediatrics* 79(1):126–127.

――――. 1983. *American Academy of Pediatrics News and Comments* 34(1):3.

――――. 1988. Age Limits of Pediatrics. A Statement by the Council on Child and Adolescent Health. *Pediatrics* 81(5):736.

――――. 1994. Policy Statement—The Role of the Non-Physician Provider in the Delivery of Pediatric Health Care. *American Academy of Pediatrics News* 10(4):22.

American Journal of Nursing. 1974. Pediatricians Withdraw Unilaterally from ANA Certification Program. 43(3):387–389.

Anders, Thomas F. 1977. Child Psychiatry and Pediatrics: The State of the Relationship. *Pediatrics* 60(4), Part 2:616–620.

Anders, Thomas F., and Michael Niehans. 1982. Promoting the Alliance Between Pediatrics and Child Psychiatry. *Pediatric Clinics of North America* 5(2):241–258.

Apple, Rima. 1980. "To Be Used Only Under the Direction of a Physician": Commercial Infant Feeding and Medical Practice. *Bulletin of the History of Medicine* 54(3):402–417.

――――. 1987. *Mothers and Medicine: A Social History of Infant Feeding, 1890–1950.* Madison, Wisconsin: University of Wisconsin Press.

Aries, Phillipe. 1962. *Centuries of Childhood: A Social History of Family Life.* New York: Vintage Books.

Arney, William R., and Bernard Bergen. 1984. *Medicine and the Management of Living: Taming the Last Great Beast.* Chicago: University of Chicago Press.

Aronson, Naomi. 1982. Nutrition as a Social Problem: A Case Study of Entrepreneurial Strategy in Science. *Social Problems* 29(5):474–487.

――――. 1984. Science as a Claims-Making Activity: Implications for Social Problems Research. Pp. 1–30 in *Studies in the Sociology of Social Problems,* edited by Joseph W. Schneider and John I. Kitsuse. Norwood, New Jersey: Ablex Publishing Company.

Atkinson, Edward R. 1985. The New Pediatrics. *American Journal of Diseases of Children* 139(4):333.

Austin, Glenn. 1975. Nurse Practitioners and School Nurses: Letter to the Editor. *Pediatrics* 54(4):620.

Backup, Molly, and John Molinaro. 1984. New Health Professionals: Changing the Hierarchy. Pp. 201–219 in *Reforming Medicine: Lessons of the Last Quarter Century,* edited by Victor Sidel and Ruth Sidel. New York: Pantheon Books.

Bass, Joel, Dorotea Johnson, Jacqueline Kirby, George A. Lamb, Janice C. Levy, Paul L. McCarthy, Carol Robins, and Cynthia Ross. 1974. Viewpoint From the Division of Community Child Health. *Pediatrics* 54(2):251.

Beaven, Paul Webley. 1955. *For the Welfare of Children: The Addresses of the First Twenty-Five Presidents of the American Academy of Pediatrics.* Springfield, Illinois: Charles C Thomas.

Becker, Howard. 1962. The Nature of a Profession. Pp. 24–46 in *Education for the Professions*, edited by the National Society for the Study of Education. Chicago: NSSE.

Bell, Susan. 1987. Changing Ideas: The Medicalization of Menopause. *Social Science and Medicine* 24(6):535–542.

Bergman, Abraham B. 1974. Pediatric Turf. *Pediatrics* 54(5):533–534.

Bergman, Abraham B., Steven W. Dassel, and Ralph J. Wedgwood. 1966. Time-Motion Study of Practicing Pediatricians. *Pediatrics* 38(2):254–263.

Best, Joel. 1987. Rhetoric in Claims-Making: Constructing the Missing Children Problem. *Social Problems* 34(2):101–121.

———. 1989a. Introduction: Typification and Social Problems Construction. Pp. xv–xxii in *Images of Issues: Typifying Contemporary Social Problems*, edited by Joel Best. New York: Aldine de Gruyter.

———. 1989b. Dark Figures and Child Victims: Statistical Claims about Missing Children. Pp. 21–37 in *Images of Issues: Typifying Social Problems*, edited by Joel Best. New York: Aldine de Gruyter.

———. 1990. *Threatened Children: Rhetoric and Concern About Child Victims*. Chicago: University of Chicago Press.

———. Ed. 1995. *Images of Issues: Typifying Contemporary Social Problems*, Second Edition. New York: Aldine de Gruyter.

Bettman, O. L. 1974. *The Good Old Days: They Were Terrible*. New York: Random House.

Billings, Dwight B., and Thomas Urban. 1982. The Socio-Medical Construction of Transsexualism: An Interpretation and Critique. *Social Problems* 29(3):266–282.

Billingsley, Molly Craig, and Doreen C. Harper. 1982. The Extinction of the Nurse Practitioner: Threat or Reality? *Nurse Practitioner* 7(October):22–30.

Birenbaum, Arnold. 1990. *In the Shadow of Medicine: Remaking the Division of Labor in Health Care*. Dix Hills, New York: General Hall.

Blim, R. Don. 1981. Report of the President. Pp. 1–2 in *Annual Report*. Evanston, Illinois: American Academy of Pediatrics.

Blumer, Herbert. 1969. *Symbolic Interactionism: Perspective and Method*. Englewood Cliffs, New Jersey: Prentice-Hall.

Bolt, Richard A. 1924. Progress in the Teaching of Preventive Pediatrics in the United States. *Transactions of the Association of American Teachers of the Diseases of Children* 18:38–47.

Boulware, J. R. 1958. The Composition of Private Pediatric Practice in a Small Community in the South of the United States: A Twenty-Five Year Survey. *Pediatrics* 22(3):548–558.

Bowers, John Z. 1976. Influences on the Development of American Medicine. Pp. 1–38 in *Advances in American Medicine*, edited by J.Z. Bowers and Elizabeth Purcell. New York: Josiah Macy Jr. Foundation.

Breese, B. B., F. A. Disney, and W. Talpey. 1966. The Nature of a Small Pediatric Group Practice. *Pediatrics* 38(2):264–277.

Breggin Peter R., and Ginger R. Breggin. 1994. *The War Against Children: The Government's Intervention into Schools, Families and Communities in Search of Medical Care for Violence*. New York: St. Martin's Press.

Bremner, Robert Hamlett, Ed. 1971. *Children and Youth in America: A Documentary*

History, Volume 2. 1866–1932. Cambridge, Massachusetts: Harvard University Press.

Brenneman, Joseph. 1933. Pediatric Psychology and the Child Guidance Movement. *Journal of Pediatrics* 2(1):1–26.

———. 1938. Periods in the Life of the American Pediatric Society—Adolescence. *Transactions of the American Pediatric Society* 50:56–67.

Breslau, Naomi. 1982. The Contribution of Pediatric Nurse Practitioners to Child Health Care. *Advances in Pediatrics* 29:387–405.

Broadhead, Robert S. 1986. Officer Ugg, Mr. Yuk, Uncle Barf . . . Ad Nausea: Controlling Poison Control, 1950–1985. *Social Problems* 33(5):424–437.

Broadhead, Robert S., and Neil J. Facchinetti. 1985. Drug Iatrogenesis and Clinical Pharmacy: The Mutual Fate of a Social Problem and a Social Movement. *Social Problems* 32(5):425–436.

Bucher, Rue. 1962. Pathology: A Study of Social Movements in a Profession. *Social Problems* 10(1):40–51.

———. 1980. *On the Natural History of Occupations*. Paper presented at the Health Care Issues in the Eighties Conference, University of Illinois, Chicago.

———. 1988. On the Natural History of Health Care Occupations. *Work and Occupations* 15(2):131–147.

Bucher, Rue, and Anselm L. Strauss. 1961. Professions in Process. *American Journal of Sociology* 66(4):325–334.

Budetti, Peter P. 1981. The Impending Pediatric "Surplus": Causes, Implications and Alternatives. *Pediatrics* 67(5):597–606.

Budetti, Peter P., John J. Frey, and Peggy McManus. 1982. Pediatricians and Family Practitioners: Future Competition for Child Patients. *Journal of Family Practice* 15(1):89–96.

Bullough, Bonnie, Harry Sultz, O. Marie Henry and Roger Fiedler. 1984. Trends in Pediatric Nurse Practitioner Education and Employment. *Pediatric Nursing* 10(May/June):193–196.

Burke, Bryan L., and Daniel P. McGee. 1990. Sports Deficit Disorder. *Pediatrics* 85(6):1118.

Butler, Colleen. 1984. The 1983 NAPNAP Membership Survey. *Pediatric Nursing* 10(May/June):187–190.

Carr, Walter Lester. 1912. The Relation of the American Pediatric Society to the Reduction of Mortality in Infancy and Childhood. *Transactions of the American Pediatric Society* 14:6–13.

Carrier, J. G. 1986. *Learning Disability: Social Class and the Construction of Inequality in American Education*. Westport, Conn.: Greenwood Press.

Casebeer, J. B. 1883. Pediatric Medicine and Its Relation to General Medicine. *Journal of the AMA* 1(9):327–330.

Castel, Robert, Francoise Castel, and Anne Lovell. 1982. *The Psychiatric Society*. New York: Columbia University Press.

Chappell, James A., and Patricia A. Drogos. 1972. Evaluation of Infant Health Care by a Nurse Practitioner. *Pediatrics* 49(6):871–877.

Charney, Evan. 1974. Forward to a Symposium on Ambulatory Pediatrics. *Pediatric Clinics of North America* 21(1):3–4.

————. 1995. The Education of Pediatricians for Primary Care: The Score After Two Score Years. *Pediatrics* 95(2):270–271.

Cleveland, William W. 1985. Dormant Correspondence Reconsidered. *Journal of Pediatrics* 107(6):910–911.

Coddington, R. Dean. 1959. Letter to the Editor. *Pediatrics* 23(5):1008.

Cohen, Michael I. 1984. The Society for Behavioral Pediatrics: A New Portal in a Rapidly Moving Boundary. *Pediatrics* 73(6):791–798.

Cohen, Ronald D. 1985. Child-Saving and Progressivism, 1885–1915. Pp. 273–309 in *American Childhood: A Research Guide and Historical Handbook*, edited by Joseph M. Hawes and N. Ray Hiner. Westport, Conn.: Greenwood Press.

Cole, Wyman C. C. 1959. Pediatrics in the Space Age. *Journal of the AMA* 171(6):641–643.

Coleman, Jules V., Donald L. Patrick, and Sidney M. Baker. 1977. The Mental Health of Children in an HMO Program. *Journal of Pediatrics* 91(4):150–153

Coltrane, Scott, and Neal Hickman. 1992. The Rhetoric of Rights and Needs: Moral Discourse in the Reform of Child Custody and Child Support Laws. *Social Problems* 39(4):400–420.

Cone, Thomas E. 1979. *History of American Pediatrics*. Boston: Little, Brown.

Conrad, Peter. 1975. The Discovery of Hyperkinesis: Notes on the Medicalization of Deviant Behavior. *Social Problems* 23(1):12–21.

————. 1976. *Identifying Hyperactive Children: The Medicalization of Deviant Behavior*. Lexington, Mass.: D. C. Heath.

————. 1992. Medicalization and Social Control. *Annual Review of Sociology* 18:209–232.

Conrad, Peter, and Joseph W. Schneider. 1980a. *Deviance and Medicalization: From Badness to Sickness*. St. Louis: C. V. Mosby.

————. 1980b. Looking at Levels of Medicalization: A Comment on Strong's Critique of the Thesis of Medical Imperialism. *Social Science and Medicine* 14(A):75–79.

Costello, Elizabeth J., Craig Edelbrock, Anthony J. Costello, Mina K. Dulcan, Barbara J. Burns, and David Brent. 1988. Psychopathology in Pediatric Primary Care: The New Hidden Morbidity. *Pediatrics* 82(3):415–424.

Coulter, Harris L. 1969. *Political and Social Aspects of 19th Century Medicine in the United States*. Ph.D. Dissertation. Department of Political Science, Columbia University, New York.

Council on Graduate Medical Education. 1988. *First Report of the Council*, Volume II. Washington D.C.: U. S. Department of Health and Human Services, Public Health Services, Health Resources and Services Administration.

Crook, William G. 1969. A Practicing Pediatrician Looks at Associates, Assistants and Aides. *Pediatric Clinics of North America* 16(4):929–938.

————. 1990. Sports Deficit Disorder. *Pediatrics* 86(5):804.

Darley, Eugene A. 1911. The Use of Whole Milk and Fat Diminished Milk in Infant Feeding. *Boston Medical and Surgical Journal* 165(20):747–754.

Davis, Starkey D. 1975. It's the Right Direction: Letter to the Editor. *Pediatrics* 56(5):840.

Davison, W. C. 1952. The Pediatric Shift. *Journal of Pediatrics* 40(4):536–538.

Day, Lewis R., Rosemarie Egli, and Henry K. Silver. 1970. Acceptance of Pediatric Nurse Practitioners. *American Journal of Diseases of Children* 119(3):204–208.

DeCastro, Fernando J., and Ursula T. Rolfe. 1974. An Evaluation of New Primary Pediatric Paraprofessionals. *Journal of Medical Education* 49(2):192–193.

Degler, Carl. 1980. *At Odds: Women and the Family in America From the Revolution to the Present.* New York: Oxford University Press.

Deisher, Robert W. 1953a. Issaquah School Health Program. *Journal of Medical Education* 28(9):26–29.

———. 1953b. Use of the Child Health Conference in the Training of Medical Students. *Pediatrics* 11(5):538–543.

———. 1955. Pediatric Residency Program. *Pediatrics* 16(4):541–543.

———. 1960. Do Education and Training Provide for the Realities of Pediatric Practice? Pp. 16–25 in *Careers in Pediatrics*, edited by Richard H. Spitz. Report of the Thirty-sixth Ross Conference on Pediatric Research. Columbus, Ohio: Ross Laboratories.

Deisher, Robert W., Alfred J. Derby, and Melvin J. Sturman. 1960. Changing Trends in Pediatric Practice. *Pediatrics* 25(4):711–716.

Diesher, Robert W., William L. Engel, Robert Spielholz, and Susan J. Standfast. 1965. Mothers' Opinion of Their Pediatric Care. *Pediatrics* 35(1):82–90.

Dubos, Rene. 1959. *The Mirage of Health.* New York: Harper & Row.

Dulles, Foster R. 1950. *The American Red Cross: A History.* New York: Harper.

Duncan, Burris, Ann N. Smith, and Henry K. Silver. 1971. Comparison of the Physical Assessment of Children by Pediatric Nurse Practitioners and Pediatricians. *American Journal of Public Health* 61(6):1170–1176.

Dworkin, Paul H., Jack P. Shonkoff, Alan Leviton, and Melvin D. Levine. 1979. Training in Developmental Pediatrics—How Practitioners Perceive the Gap. *American Journal of Diseases of Children* 133(7):709–712.

Dye, Nancy Schrom, and Daniel Blake Smith. 1986. Mother Love and Infant Death, 1750–1920. *Journal of American History* 73(2):329–353.

Eaton, Antoinette Parisi. 1991. What Happened to the Predicted Glut of Pediatricians? *Pediatrics* 88(4):870–871.

Ehrenreich, Barbara, and Deirdre English. 1979. *For Her Own Good: 150 Years of Experts' Advice to Women.* Garden City, New York: Anchor Press.

Eisenberg, Leon. 1967. The Relationship Between Psychiatry and Pediatrics: A Disputatious View. *Pediatrics* 39(5):645–647.

Erchak, Gerald M., and Richard Rosenfeld. 1989. Learning Disabilities, Dyslexia, and the Medicalization of the Classroom. Pp. 79–97 in *Images of Issues: Typifying Contemporary Social Problems*, edited by Joel Best. New York: Aldine de Gruyter.

Etzioni, Amitai. 1964. *Modern Organizations.* Englewood Cliffs, New Jersey: Prentice-Hall.

Evans, Philip R. 1967. Fashions in Infant Feeding. Pp. 307–317 in *A Symposium on the Child*, edited by J. A. Askin, R. E. Cooke, and J. A. Haller, Jr. Baltimore: Johns Hopkins Press.

Faber, Harold K., and Rustin McIntosh. 1966. *History of the American Pediatric Society, 1887–1965.* New York: McGraw-Hill.

Figert, Anne E. 1995. The Three Faces of PMS: The Professional, Gendered, and Scientific Structuring of a Psychiatric Disorder. *Social Problems* 42(1):56–73.

Finkelstein, Barbara. 1985. Casting Networks of Good Influence: The Reconstruction of Childhood in the United States, 1790–1870. Pp. 111–152 in *American Childhood: A Research Guide and Historical Handbook* edited by Joseph M. Hawes and N. Ray Hiner. Westport, Conn.: Greenwood Press.

Fischer, Carl C. 1957. The Pediatrician and His Changing World. *Journal of Pediatrics* 51(5):593–605.

Fishman, Daniel B., and C. N. Zimet. 1972. Specialty Choice and Beliefs About Specialties Among Freshman Medical Students. *Journal of Medical Education* 47(7):524–533.

Folsom, Marion B. 1966. *Health Is a Community Affair*. Report of the National Commission on Community Health Services. Cambridge, Mass.: Harvard University Press.

Ford, Loretta C. 1979. A Nurse for all Settings: The Nurse Practitioner. *Nursing Outlook* 27(8):516–521.

————. 1982. Nurse Practitioners: History of a New Idea and Predictions for the Future. Pp. 231–247 in *Nursing in the 1980s: Crises, Opportunities, Challenges*, edited by Linda H. Aiken. Philadelphia: J. B. Lippincott.

Freidson, Eliot. 1970a. *Profession of Medicine: A Study of the Sociology of Applied Knowledge*. New York: Dodd, Mead.

————. 1970b. *Professional Dominance: The Social Structure of Medical Care*. New York: Atherton.

Friedman, Stanford B. 1970. The Challenge of Behavioral Pediatrics. *Journal of Pediatrics* 77(1):172–173.

Friedman, Stanford B., Sheridan Phillips, and John M. Parrish. 1983. Current Status of Behavioral Pediatric Training for General Pediatric Residents: A Study of Eleven Funded Programs. *Pediatrics* 71(6):904–908.

Fulginiti, Vincent A. 1987. The Future of Pediatrics: Again. *Journal of the AMA* 258(2):247–248.

Gallagher, J. Roswell. 1954. A Clinic for Adolescents. *Children* 1(5):165–170.

Gallagher, J. Roswell. 1982. The Origins, Development and Goals of Adolescent Medicine. *Journal of Adolescent Health Care* 3(1):57–63.

Garfunkel, Joseph M. 1985. The Pediatrician of the Future. *Journal of Pediatrics* 107(6):911–912.

Gee, Helen H. 1960. Characteristics of Individuals Who Select Careers in Pediatrics. Pp. 37–46 in *Careers in Pediatrics*, edited by Richard H. Spitz. Report of the Thirty-sixth Ross Conference on Pediatric Research. Columbus, Ohio: Ross Laboratories.

Gentry, Cynthia. 1988. The Social Construction of Abducted Children as a Social Problem. *Sociological Inquiry* 58(4):413–425.

Geppert, Leo J. 1958. Composition of Pediatric Practice at a Permanent Army Base in the Antibiotic Era. *Pediatrics* 22(2):336–363.

Gerber, Jurg, and James R. Short. 1984. Marketing Baby Formula as a Social Problem: The Rise, Decline and Institutionalization of a Social Movement. Paper presented at the Meetings of the Society for the Study of Social Problems. Washington, D.C.

Geyman, John P. 1971. *The Modern Family Doctor and Changing Medical Practice*. New York: Appleton, Century, Crofts.

————. 1978. Family Practice in Evolution: Progress, Problems and Projections. *New England Journal of Medicine* 298(11):593–601.

————. 1985. *Foundation of Changing Health Care*, Second Edition. Norwalk, Conn.: Appleton-Century-Crofts.

Gillespie, Dair L., and Ann Leffler. 1987. The Politics of Research Methodology in Claims-Making Activities: Social Science and Sexual Harrassment. *Social Problems* 34(5):490–501.

Gittings, John C. 1928. Pediatrics of One Hundred Years Ago. *American Journal of Diseases of Children* 36(1):1–15.

Glaser, Barney, and Anselm Strauss. 1967. *The Discovery of Grounded Theory: Strategies for Qualitative Research*. Chicago: Aldine.

Goffman, Erving. 1983. The Interaction Order: 1982 ASA Presidential Address. *American Sociological Review* 48(1):1–17.

Goldberg, Irving D., Darrel A. Regier, Thomas K. McInerny, Ivan B. Pless, and Klaus Roghmann. 1979. The Role of the Pediatrician in the Delivery of Mental Health Services to Children. *Pediatrics* 63(6):898–909.

Golden, Janet. 1989. *Infant Asylums and Children's Hospitals: Medical Dilemmas and Development, 1850–1920: An Anthology of Sources*. New York: Garland.

Gorwitz, Kurt, and Donald. C. Smith. 1975. Some Implications of Declining Birth Rates for Pediatrics. *Pediatrics* 56(4):592–597.

Gould, Kenneth S. 1964. Letter to the Editor. *Pediatrics* 33(5):789–791.

Gray, Herman. 1989. Popular Music as a Social Problem: A Social History of Claims Against Popular Music. Pp. 143–158 in *Images of Issues: Typifying Contemporary Social Problems*, edited by Joel Best. New York: Aldine de Gruyter.

Green, Morris, and Milton J. E. Senn. 1958. Teaching of Comprehensive Pediatrics on an Inpatient Service in Pediatrics. *Pediatrics* 21(3):476–490.

Green, Morris, and Mary Stark. 1957. A Postgraduate Program for the Longitudinal Health Supervision of Infants. *Pediatrics* 19(2):499–503.

Griffith, J. P. Crozer. 1898. The Rise, Progress and Present Needs of Pediatrics. *Journal of the American Medical Association* 31(17):947–951.

————. 1936. History and Recollections of the Development of Pediatrics in Philadelphia. *Pennsylvania Medical Journal* 39(8):597–603.

Gusfield, Joseph R. 1975. Categories of Ownership and Responsibility in Social Issues: Alcohol Abuse and Automobile Use. *Journal of Drug Issues* 5(Fall):285–303.

————. 1981. *The Culture of Public Problems: Drinking, Driving and the Symbolic Order*. Chicago: University of Chicago Press.

————. 1984. On the Side: Practical Action and Social Constructivism in Social Problems Theory. Pp. 31–51 in *Studies in the Sociology of Social Problems*, edited by Joseph W. Schneider and John I. Kitsuse. Norwood, N.J.: Ablex.

————. 1985. Theories and Hobgoblins. *SSSP Newsletter* 17(Fall):16–18.

Habenstein, Robert W. 1970. Occupational Uptake: Professionalizing. Pp. 99–121 in *Pathways to Data: Field Methods for Studying Ongoing Social Organizations*, edited by Robert W. Habenstein. Chicago: Aldine.

Haggerty, Robert J. 1972. Do We Really Need More Pediatricians? *Pediatrics* 50(5):681–683.

——. 1974. The Changing Role of the Pediatrician in Child Health Care. *American Journal of Diseases of Children* 127(4):545–549.

——. 1982. Behavioral Pediatrics: Can It Be Taught? Can It Be Practiced? *Pediatric Clinics of North America* 29(2):391–398.

——. 1988. Behavioral Pediatrics: A Time for Research. *Pediatrics* 81(2):179–185.

——. 1990. The Academic Generalist: An Endangered Species Revisited. *Pediatrics* 86(3):413–420.

——. 1995. Child Health 2000: New Pediatrics in the Changing Environment of Children's Needs in the 21st Century. *Pediatrics* 96(4) Supplement:804–812.

Haggerty, Robert J., Klaus J. Roghmann, and Ivan B. Pless. 1975. *Child Health and the Community*. New York: Wiley.

Halpern, Sydney. 1982. *Segmental Professionalization Within Medicine: The Case of Pediatrics*. Ph.D. Dissertation. Department of Sociology, University of California, Berkeley.

——. 1988. *American Pediatrics: The Social Dynamics of Professionalization, 1880–1980*. Berkeley: University of California Press.

——. 1990. Medicalization as Professional Process: Postwar Trends in Pediatrics. *Journal of Health and Social Behavior* 31(1):28–42.

Harned, Herbert S., Jr. 1959. A Challenge to Practitioners. *Pediatrics* 24(5):859–862.

Haug, Marie. 1973. Deprofessionalization: An Alternative Hypothesis for the Future. *Sociological Review Monographs* 20:195–211.

Hawes, Joseph M., and N. Ray Hiner. Eds. 1985. *American Childhood: A Research Guide and Historical Handbook*. Westport, Conn.: Greenwood Press.

Hazelrigg, Lawrence E. 1985. Were It Not For Words. *Social Problems* 32(3):234–237.

Herman, Mary W., and Jon Veloski. 1977. Family Medicine and Primary Care: Trends and Student Characteristics. *Journal of Medical Education* 5(22):99–106.

Hess, Julius H. 1917. The Pediatric Curriculum as Taught in the Class "A" Medical Schools in the United States. *Transactions of the Association of American Teachers of Diseases of Children* 11:22–25.

Hessel, Samuel J., and Robert J. Haggerty. 1968. General Pediatrics: A Study of Practice in the Mid-1960s. *Journal of Pediatrics* 73(2):271–279.

Hick, John F. 1970. The Young Male Prostitute—A Letter to the Editor. *Pediatrics* 45(1):153–154.

Hickson, Gerald B., William A. Altemeir, and Susan O'Connor. 1983. Concerns of Mothers Seeking Care in Private Pediatric Offices: Opportunities for Expanding Services. *Pediatrics* 72(5):619–624.

Hill, Lee Forest. 1957. Correspondence. *Journal of Pediatrics* 51(6):747.

——. 1960. Anticipatory Guidance in Pediatric Practice. *Journal of Pediatrics* 56(2):299–307.

Hoekelman, Robert A. 1981. Forward. Pp. xiii–xv in *Behavioral Problems in Child-*

hood: A Primary Care Approach, edited by Stewart Gabel. New York: Grune & Stratton.

Hoekelman, Robert A., Michael Klein, and James E. Strain. 1984. Who Should Provide Primary Health Care to Children: Pediatricians or Family Medicine Physicians? *Pediatrics* 74(4):460–477.

Holstein, James A., and Gale Miller, Eds. 1993. *Reconsidering Constructionism: Debates in Social Problems Theory*. New York: Aldine de Gruyter.

Holt, L. Emmett. 1923. American Pediatrics—A Retrospect and a Forecast: President's Address. *Transactions of the American Pediatric Society* 35:9–17.

Holt, L. Emmett, Jr. 1961. Pediatrics at the Delta: Presidential Address to the American Pediatric Society. *American Journal of Diseases of Children* 102 (11):671–676.

Hubbell, John P. 1989. Review of *American Pediatrics: The Social Dynamics of Professionalism, 1880–1980* by Sydney Halpern. *New England Journal of Medicine* 320(20):1357–1358.

Hughes, Everett C. 1951. Work and Self. Pp. 313–323 in *Social Psychology at the Crossroads*, edited by J. H. Rohrer and Muzafer Sherif. New York: Harper & Row.

———. 1961. Education for a Profession. *Library Quarterly* 31(4):336–343.

———. 1971. *The Sociological Eye: Selected Papers on Work, Self and the Study of Society*. Chicago: Aldine.

Hughes, James G. 1980. *American Academy of Pediatrics: The First 50 Years*. Evanston, Illinois: The American Academy of Pediatrics.

Ibarra, Peter R., and John I. Kitsuse. 1993. Vernacular Constituents of Moral Discourse: An Interactionist Proposal for the Study of Social Problems. Pp. 21–54 in *Constructionist Controversies: Issues in Social Problems Theory*, edited by Gale Miller and James A. Holstein. New York: Aldine de Gruyter.

Illich, Ivan. 1976. *Limits to Medicine, Medical Nemesis: The Expropriation of Health*. London: Marion Boyars.

Jacobi, Abraham. 1889. The Relation of Pediatrics to General Medicine: President's Address. *Transactions of the American Pediatric Society* 1:6–17.

———. 1908. The Gospel of the Top Milk. *Journal of the AMA* 51 (15):1216–1219.

Jacobziner, Harold, Herbert Rich, and Roland Mercant. 1962. Pediatric Care in Private Practice. *Journal of the AMA* 182(10):986–993.

Jenness, Valerie. 1993. *Making It Work: The Prostitutes' Rights Movement in Perspective*. New York: Aldine de Gruyter.

Johnson, John M. 1989. Horror Stories and the Construction of Child Abuse. Pp. 5–19 in *Images of Issues: Typifying Contemporary Social Problems*, edited by Joel Best. New York: Aldine de Gruyter.

Johnson, Michael P., and Karl Hufbauer. 1982. Sudden Infant Death Syndrome as a Medical and Research Problem since 1945. *Social Problems* 30(1):65–81.

Jones, Kathleen W. 1983. Sentiment and Science: The Late Nineteenth Century Pediatrician as Mother's Advisor. *Journal of Social History* 17(Fall):79–95.

Journal of the AMA. 1891. Pediatrics. 17(October):603–604.

———. 1980. Medical Education in the United States: 1979–1980. 244(25):2801–2871.

―――. 1982. Medical Education in the United States: 1981–1982. 248(24):3223–3293.

―――. 1984. Medical Education in the United States: 1983–1984. 252(12):1515–1633.

―――. 1985. Medical Education in the United States: 1984–1985. 254(12):1545–1658.

―――. 1986. Medical Education in the United States: 1985–1986. 256(12):1545–1662.

Kahn, Lawrence. 1979. The Influence of Funding on the Future of PNP Programs in Pediatrics. *Pediatrics* 64(1):106–110.

Katcher, Ayrum L. 1974. Dr. Nathan's Assumptions Attacked. *Pediatrics* 54(2):251.

Kempe, C. Henry. 1978. The 1978 Presidential Address to the American Pediatric Society: The Future of Pediatrics. *Pediatric Research* 12(12):1149–1151.

King, Charles R. 1993. *Children's Health in America: A History.* New York: Twayne Publishers.

Kirk, Stuart A., and Herb Kutchins. 1992. *The Selling of DSM: The Rhetoric of Science in Psychiatry.* New York: Aldine de Gruyter.

Kitsuse, John I. 1980. Coming Out All Over: Deviants and the Politics of Social Problems. *Social Problems* 28:1–13.

Kitsuse, John I., and A. Cicourel. 1963. A Note on the Use of Official Statistics. *Social Problems* 11(2):131–139.

Korsch, Barbara M. 1960. Qualitative and Quantitative Components of a Pediatric Practitioner's Education and Training. Pp. 37–46 in *Careers in Pediatrics,* edited by Richard M. Spitz. Report of the Thirty-Sixth Ross Conference on Pediatric Research. Columbus, Ohio: Ross Laboratories.

Korsch, Barbara M., Francis Negrete Vida, Ann S. Mercer, and Barbara Freemon. 1971. How Comprehensive Are Well-Child Visits? *American Journal of Diseases of Children* 122(12):483–488.

Kotch, Jonathan B. 1976. Pediatrics: The End or the Beginning? *American Academy of Pediatrics News and Comments* 27(12):9–11.

LaFetra, L. E. 1932. The Development of Pediatrics in New York City. *Archives of Pediatrics* 49(1):36–60.

Lasch, Christopher. 1979. *Haven in a Heartless World: The Family Besieged.* New York: Basic Books.

Laslett, Barbara. 1978. Family Membership, Past and Present. *Social Problems* 25(5):476–490.

Lawson, Robert B. 1960. Historical Perspectives on Pediatrics in the United States. Pp. 14–16 in *Careers in Pediatrics,* edited by Robert H. Spitz. Report of the Thirty-sixth Ross Conference on Pediatric Research. Columbus, Ohio: Ross Laboratories.

Levine, Samuel Z. 1960. Pediatric Education at the Crossroads: Presidential Address to the American Pediatric Society. *American Journal of Diseases of Children* 100(11):651–656.

Lewis, Charles E. 1982. Nurse Practitioners and the Physician Surplus. Pp. 249–

266 in *Nursing in the 1980s: Crises, Opportunities, Challenges*, edited by Linda H. Aiken. Philadelphia: J. B. Lippincott.

London, Arthur H. 1937. The Composition of an Average Pediatric Practice. *Journal of Pediatrics* 10(6):762–771.

Low, Merritt B. 1977. Presidential Address—1976: Whither Pediatrics. *Pediatrics* 59(4):499–504.

Lucas, William Palmer. 1927. *The Modern Practice of Pediatrics*. New York: Macmillan.

MacQueen, John C. 1975. *Presidential Address*. Read before the Meetings of the American Academy of Pediatrics. Washington, D.C.

Margolin, Leslie. 1994. *Goodness Personified: The Emergence of Gifted Children*. New York: Aldine de Gruyter.

Mathieu, Owen R., and Joel J. Alpert. 1987. Residency Training in General Pediatrics. *American Journal of Diseases of Children* 141(7):754–757.

Maurer, Donna, and Jeffery Sobal. Eds. 1995. *Eating Agendas: Food and Nutrition as Social Problems*. New York: Aldine de Gruyter.

May, Charles D. 1959. Can the New Pediatrics Be Practiced? *Pediatrics* 23(2):253–254.

———. 1960. The Future of Pediatricians as Medical Specialists. *American Journal of Diseases of Children* 100(11):661–668.

McAnarney, Elizabeth R. 1986. Pediatrics to Geriatrics? *American Journal of Diseases of Children* 140(9):866.

McCleary, G. F. 1933. *The Early History of the Infant Welfare Movement*. London: H. K. Lewis.

McCranie, E. W., J. L. Hornsby, and J. C. Cavert. 1982. Practice and Career Satisfaction Among Residents Trained in Family Practice. *Journal of Family Practice* 14(6):1107–1114.

McCrea, Francis B. 1983. The Politics of Menopause: The "Discovery" of a Deficiency Disease. *Social Problems* 31(1):111–123.

McCune, Yolanda D., Miriam M. Richardson, and Judith A. Powell. 1984. Psychosocial Health Issues in Pediatric Practices: Parents' Knowledge and Concerns. *Pediatrics* 74(2):183–190.

McKeown, Thomas. 1979. *The Role of Medicine: Dream, Mirage, or Nemesis?* Princeton, N.J.: Princeton University Press.

McKinlay, John B., and Sonja J. McKinlay. 1977. The Questionable Effect of Medical Measures on the Decline of Mortality in the United States in the Twentieth Century. *Milbank Memorial Fund Quarterly* 55:405–428.

Mead, George Herbert. 1934. *Mind, Self and Society*. Chicago: University of Chicago Press.

Medical Economics. 1956. Medicine's Most Frustrating Specialty. 33(November):68–74.

———. 1961. How the Specialties Compare Financially. 38(March):88–93.

Miller, Gale, and James A. Holstein. Eds. 1993. *Constructionist Controversies: Issues in Social Problems Theory*. New York: Aldine de Gruyter.

Millerson, Geoffrey. 1964. *The Qualifying Associations: A Study in Professionalization*. London: Routledge and Kegan Paul.

Millis, J. S. Chairman. 1966. *The Graduate Education of Physicians*. Report of the Citizens' Commission on Graduate Medical Education. Chicago: American Medical Association.

Moloney, Margaret M. 1986. *Professionalization of Nursing: Current Issues and Trends*. Philadelphia: J.B. Lippincott.

Morrow, Carol Klaperman. 1982. Sick Doctors: The Social Construction of Professional Deviance. *Social Problems* 30(1):92–108.

Morse, John Lovett. 1935. Recollections and Reflections on Forty-five Years of Artificial Feeding. *Journal of Pediatrics* 7(3):303–324.

———. 1937. The Future of Pediatrics. *Journal of Pediatrics* 10(4):529–532.

Musgrove, Frank. 1964. *Youth and the Social Order*. London: Routledge and Kegan Paul.

Nadler, Henry L., and Wendy J. Evans. 1987. The Future of Pediatrics. *American Journal of Diseases of Children* 141(1):21–27.

Nathan, David G. 1973. Primary Medical Care and Medical Research Training. *Pediatrics* 52(6):768–772.

Nelson, Waldo E. 1955. Trends in Pediatrics. *Journal of Pediatrics* 47(1):109–123.

Oates, Richard P., and Harry A. Feldman. 1974. Patterns of Change in Medical Student Career Choices. *Journal of Medical Education* 49(6):562–569.

Official American Board of Medical Specialists Directory of Board Certified Medical Specialists—1995, 27th Edition. 1994. New Providence, New Jersey: Marquis Who's Who. A Reed Reference Publishing Company.

Olmsted, Richard W. 1978. Pediatrics: A Perspective on the Present and Future of a Proud Profession. *American Journal of Diseases of Children* 132(10):962–966.

———. 1979. A Perspective: Pediatrics Today and Tomorrow. *American Academy of Pediatrics News and Comments* 30(8):9–11.

Ott, John E. 1975. New Health Professionals in Pediatrics. *Advances in Pediatrics* 20(1):39–67.

Park, Edward A., and Howard H. Mason. 1957. Luther Emmett Holt. Pp. 33–60 in *Pediatric Profiles*, edited by Borden S. Veeder. St. Louis: C. V. Mosby.

Parton, Nigel. 1979. A Natural History of Child Abuse: A Study in Social Problem Definition. *British Journal of Social Work* 9(4):431–451.

Patterson, Patricia K., Abraham B. Bergman, and R. J. Wedgwood. 1969. Parent Reaction to the Concept of Pediatric Assistants. *Pediatrics* 44(1):69–75.

Pawluch, Dorothy. 1996. Social Problems. Pp. 797–799 in *The Social Science Encyclopedia*, Second Edition, edited by Adam Kuper and Jessica Kuper. London: Routledge.

Pearson, Howard A. 1988. *The Centennial History of the American Pediatric Society, 1888–1988*. New Haven, Connecticut: Yale University Printing Service.

———. 1991. Pediatrics in the United States. Pp. 55–63 in *History of Pediatrics, 1850–1950*, edited by Buford L. Nichols, Jr., Angel Ballabriga, and Norman Kretchmer. Nestle Nutrition Workshop Series, Vol. 22. New York: Raven Press.

———. 1995. The American Pediatric Society. *Pediatrics* 95(1):147–151.

Pease, Marshall Carleton. 1951. *A History of the American Academy of Pediatrics—June 1930 to June 1951*. Evanston, Illinois: The American Academy of Pediatrics.

Pellegrino, Edmund. 1978. The Academic Viability of Family Medicine. *Journal of the AMA* 240(2):132–135.

Pfohl, Stephen. 1977. The "Discovery" of Child Abuse. *Social Problems* 24(3):310–324.

———. 1985. Toward a Sociological Deconstruction of Social Problems. *Social Problems* 32(3):228–232.

———. 1994. *Images of Deviance and Social Control: A Sociological History*. Second Edition. New York: McGraw-Hill.

Pfundt, Theodore R. 1961. A Retrospective Residency Evaluation by Practicing Pediatricians. *Journal of Medical Education* 36(5):414–417.

Platt, Anthony. 1969. *The Child Savers: The Invention of Delinquency*. Chicago: University of Chicago Press.

Pless, Ivan B. 1974. The Changing Face of Primary Pediatrics. *Pediatric Clinics of North America* 21(1):223–244.

Posner, Michael K. 1974. Are the Academicians to Blame? *Pediatrics* 54(2):249.

Powers, Grover F. 1955. American Pediatrics: The Coming Years. *Pediatrics* 16(5):688–694.

Preston, Samuel H., and Michael R. Haines. 1991. *Fatal Years: Child Mortality in Late Nineteenth-Century America*. Princeton, New Jersey: Princeton University Press.

Prugh, Dane G. 1983. *The Psychosocial Aspects of Pediatrics*. Philadelphia: Lea & Febiger.

Pyeritz, Reed E. 1974. Intellectual Elitism Attacked. *Pediatrics* 54(2):249–250.

Rafter, Nicole H. 1992. Some Consequences of Strict Constructionism. *Social Problems* 39(1):38–39.

Reed, James. 1978. *From Private Vice to Public Virtue: The Birth Control Movement and American Society Since 1830*. New York: Basic Books.

Reisinger, Keith S., and Jill A. Bires. 1980. Anticipatory Guidance in Pediatric Practice. *Pediatrics* 66(6):889–892.

Richmond, Julius B. 1959. Some Observations on the Sociology of Pediatric Education and Practice. *Pediatrics* 23(6):1175–1178.

———. 1967. Child Development: A Basic Science for Pediatrics. *Pediatrics* 39(5):649–657.

———. 1975. An Idea Whose Time Has Arrived. *Pediatric Clinics of North America* 22(3):517–523.

Richmond, Julius B., and Juel M. Janis. 1983. Ripeness Is All: The Coming of Age of Behavioral Pediatrics. Pp. 15–23 in *Developmental-Behavioral Pediatrics*, edited by Melvin D. Levine, William B. Carey, Allen C. Crocker, and Ruth T. Gross. Philadelphia: W. B. Saunders.

Riessman, Catherine Kohler. 1983. Women and Medicalization: A New Perspective. *Social Policy* 14(Summer):3–18.

Riessman, Catherine Kohler, and Constance A. Nathanson. 1986. The Management of Reproduction: Social Construction of Risk and Responsibility. Pp. 251–281 in *Applications of Social Science to Clinical Medicine and Health Policy*, edited by Linda H. Aiken and David Mechanic. New Brunswick, New Jersey: Rutgers University Press.

Ritzer, George, and David Walczak. 1986. *Working: Conflict and Change*, Third Edition. Englewood Cliffs, N.J.: Prentice-Hall.

Robbins, Thomas, and Dick Anthony. 1982. Deprogramming, Brainwashing and the Medicalization of Deviant Religious Groups. *Social Problems* 29(3):283–297.

Rogers, David E., Robert J. Blendon, and Ruby P. Hearn. 1981. Some Observations on Pediatrics: Its Past, Present and Future. *Pediatrics* 67(5) Supplement:776–784.

Rogers, Kenneth D. 1960. A Teaching Program in Community Pediatrics. *Pediatrics* 25(2):336–339.

Rogers, Martha. 1972. Nursing: To Be or Not to Be. *Nursing Outlook* 20(1):42–45.

Rose, John A., and Donald C. Ross. 1960. Comprehensive Pediatrics: Postgraduate Training for Practicing Physicians. *Pediatrics* 25(1):135–144.

Rose, Vicki McNickle. 1977. Rape as a Social Problem: A Byproduct of the Feminist Movement. *Social Problems* 25(1):75–89.

Rosecrance, John. 1985. Compulsive Gambling and the Medicalization of Deviance. *Social Problems* 32(3):275–284.

Rosen, George. [1958] 1993. *A History of Public Health*. Baltimore, Maryland: Johns Hopkins University Press.

———. 1975. *Preventive Medicine in the United States, 1900–1975: Trends and Interpretations*. New York: Science History Publications.

Rosenberg, Charles E. 1983. Prologue: The Shape of Traditional Practice, 1800–1875. Pp. 1–12 in *The Structure of American Medical Practice, 1875–1941*, edited by George Rosen. Philadelphia: University of Pennsylvania Press.

Rosengren, William R. 1980. *Sociology of Medicine: Diversity, Conflict and Change*. New York: Harper & Row.

Rosinski, E. F., and F. Dagenais. 1978. *Resident Training for Primary Care: A Study of Nine Residency Programs Supported by the Robert Wood Johnson Foundation*. San Francisco: University of California.

Rotch, Thomas Morgan. 1891. Iconoclasm and Original Thought in the Study of Pediatrics: President's Address. *Transactions of the American Pediatric Society* 3:6–9.

———. 1903. *Pediatrics*. Fourth Edition. Philadelphia: Lippincott.

Roth, Julius A. 1974. Professionalism: The Sociologist's Decoy. *Sociology of Work and Occupations* 1(1):6–23.

Sarbin, T. R., and John I. Kitsuse. 1994. A Prologue to Constructing Social Problems. Pp. 1–18 in *Constructing the Social*, edited by T. R Sarbin and John I. Kitsuse. Thousand Oaks, California: Sage.

Schiff, Donald W., Charles H. Fraser, and Heather L. Walters. 1969. The Pediatric Nurse Practitioner in the Office of Pediatricians in Private Practice. *Pediatrics* 44(1):62–68.

Schlutz, Frederic W. 1933. First Half Century of the Section on Pediatrics. *Journal of the AMA* 101(5):417–420.

Schmitt, Barton D. 1969. Responsibility for School Problems: An Objection to "Pediatric Globalism." *Pediatrics* 44(5):771–772.

Schneider, Joseph. 1978. Deviant Drinking as Disease: Alcoholism as Social Accomplishment. *Social Problems* 25(4):361–372.

————. 1985a. Social Problems Theory: The Constructionist View. *Annual Review of Sociology* II:209–229.

————. 1985b. Defining the Definitional Perspective on Social Problems. *Social Problems* 32(3):232–234.

Schneider, Joseph, and John I. Kitsuse. 1984. *Studies in the Sociology of Social Problems*. Norwood, N.J.: Ablex.

Schumacher, Charles F. 1964. Personal Characteristics of Students Choosing Different Types of Medical Careers. *Journal of Medical Education* 39(3):278–288.

Schwartz, Howard D., Peggy L. de Wolf, and James K. Skipper, Jr. 1987. Gender, Professionalization and Occupational Anomie: The Case of Nursing. Pp. 559–569 in *Dominant Issues in Medical Sociology*, Second Edition, edited by Howard D. Schwartz. New York: Random House.

Scott, Wilbur J. 1990. PTSD in DSM-III: A Case in the Politics of Diagnosis and Disease. *Social Problems* 37(3):294–310.

Scritchfield, Shirley A. 1989. The Social Construction of Infertility: From Private Matter to Social Concern. Pp. 99–114 in *Images of Issues: Typifying Contemporary Social Problems*, edited by Joel Best. New York: Aldine de Gruyter.

Sedgwick, Peter. 1973. Illness—Mental and Otherwise. *Hastings Center Studies* 1(3):19–40.

Senn, Milton J. E. 1956. An Orientation for Instruction in Pediatrics. *Journal of Medical Education* 31(9):613–619.

Sharp, Lee, Robert H. Pantell, Lisa O. Murphy, and Catherine C. Lewis. 1992. Psychosocial Problems During Child Health Supervision Visits: Eliciting, Then What? *Pediatrics* 89(4):619–623.

Shiller, Jack G. 1974. Training Pediatricians for Primary Medical Care. *Pediatrics* 54(2):131–132.

Shrag, Peter, and Diane Divoky. 1975. *The Myth of the Hyperactive Child*. New York: Dell.

Shryock, Richard H. 1936. *The Development of Modern Medicine*. Madison: University of Wisconsin Press.

Sills, David L. 1957. *The Volunteers*. Glencoe, Illinois: The Free Press.

Silver, George A. 1963. Family Practice: Resuscitation or Reform? *Journal of the AMA* 185(3):188–191.

Silver, Henry K. 1968. Use of New Types of Allied Health Professionals in Providing Care for Children. *American Journal of Diseases of Children* 116(11):486–490.

Silver, Henry K., Loretta C. Ford, and Susan G. Stearly. 1967. A Program to Increase Health Care for Children: The Pediatric Nurse Practitioner Program. *Pediatrics* 39(5):756–760.

Sklar, June, and Beth Berkov. 1974. Abortion, Illegitimacy and the American Birth Rate. *Science* 185(4155):909–915.

Smillie, W. G. 1955. *Public Health, Its Promise for the Future*. New York: Macmillan.

Smith, David H., and Robert A. Hoekelman. 1981. *Controversies in Child Health and Pediatric Practice*. New York: McGraw-Hill.

Solnit, Albert J., and Milton J. E. Senn. 1954. Teaching Comprehensive Pediatrics in an Out-Patient Clinic. *Pediatrics* 14(5):547–556.

Spector, Malcolm. 1977. Legitimizing Homosexuality. *Society* 14(5):52–56.
Spector, Malcolm, and John I. Kitsuse. [1977] 1987. *Constructing Social Problems.* New York: Aldine de Gruyter.
Spitz, Richard H., Ed. 1960. *Careers in Pediatrics.* Report of the Thirty-sixth Ross Conference on Pediatric Research. Columbus, Ohio: Ross Laboratories.
Stafford, Henry E. 1936. The Changing Pediatric Practice. *Journal of Pediatrics* 8(3):375–380.
Stallings, Robert A. 1995. *Promoting Risk: Constructing the Earthquake Threat.* New York: Aldine de Gruyter.
Stannard, David E. 1977. *The Puritan Way of Death.* New York: Oxford University Press.
Starfield, Barbara. 1982. Behavioral Pediatrics and Primary Health Care. *Pediatric Clinics of North America* 29(2):377–390.
———. 1983. Special Responsibilities: The Role of the Pediatrician and the Goals of Pediatric Education. *Pediatrics* 71(3):433–440.
Starfield, Barbara, and Shirley Borkowf. 1969. Physicians' Recognition of Complaints Made By Parents About Their Children's Health. *Pediatrics* 43(2):168–172.
Starfield, Barbara, Edward Gross, Maurice Wood, Robert Pantell, Constance Allen, I. Bruce Gordon, Patricia Moffat, Robert Drachman, and Harvey Katz. 1980. Psychosocial and Psychosomatic Diagnoses in Primary Care of Children. *Pediatrics* 66(2):159–167.
Starfield, Barbara, and E. Sharp. 1971. Medical Problems, Medical Care, and School Performance. *Journal of School Health* 41(2):184–187.
Starr, Paul. 1982. *The Social Transformation of American Medicine.* New York: Basic Books.
Stehbens, James A., and R. M. Lauer. 1972. Pediatric Cardiology: A New Role for the Pediatric Assistant. *Journal of Pediatrics* 81(2):394–398.
Stevens, Rosemary. 1971. *American Medicine and the Public Interest.* New Haven, Connecticut: Yale University Press.
Stewart, William H. 1967. The Unmet Needs of Children. *Pediatrics* 39(2):157–160.
Stewart, William, and Maryland Y. Pennel. 1963. Pediatric Manpower in the United States and Its Implications. *Pediatrics* 31(2):311–318.
St. Geme, Joseph W., Jr. 1981. Let's Speak Up For Pediatricians. *Pediatrics* 68(5):734–735.
Stone, Lawrence. 1977. *The Family, Sex and Marriage in England, 1500–1800.* New York: Harper & Row.
Strain, James E. 1983. Pediatrician's Role in Primary Health Care. *Pediatrics* 71(3):441–442.
Straus, Robert. 1957. The Nature and Status of Medical Sociology. *American Sociological Review* 22(2):200–204.
Strong, P. M. 1979. Sociological Imperialism and the Profession of Medicine: A Critical Examination of the Thesis of Medical Imperialism. *Social Science and Medicine* 13(2):199–213.
Tabrah, Frank L. 1957. Letter to the Editor. *Journal of Pediatrics* 51(6):745–747.

Talbot, Nathan B. 1960. "The New Pediatrics" and Medical Education. *Journal of Medical Education* 35(10):913–915.

Talbat, Nathan B. 1963. Has Psychological Malnutrition Taken the Place of Rickets and Scurvy in Contemporary Pediatric Practice? *Pediatrics* 31(6):909–918.

Task Force on Pediatric Education. 1978. *The Future of Pediatric Education.* Evanston, Illinois: American Academy of Pediatrics.

Thompson, Hugh C. 1984. 20th Century U.S. Child Health Care: Past, Present, Future. *American Journal of Diseases of Children* 138(9):804–809.

Tierney, Kathleen J. 1982. The Battered Women Movement and the Creation of the Wife Beating Problem. *Social Problems* 29(3):207–220.

Tiffin, Susan. 1982. *In Whose Best Interest? Child Welfare Reform in the Progressive Era.* Westport, Conn.: Greenwood Press.

Toister, R. P., and L. M. Worley. 1976. Behavioral Aspects of Pediatric Practice: A Survey of Practitioners. *Journal of Medical Education* 51(12):1019–1020.

Tompkins, Charles A. 1959. Letter to the Editor. *Pediatrics* 23(5):1013–1015.

Troyer, Ronald J. 1989. The Surprising Resurgence of the Smoking Problem. Pp. 159–176 in *Images of Issues: Typifying Contemporary Social Problems,* edited by Joel Best. New York: Aldine de Gruyter.

———. 1992. Some Consequences of Contextual Constructionism. *Social Problems* 39(1):35–37.

UNICEF. 1990. *Children and Development in the 1990s: A UNICEF Sourcebook.* New York: UNICEF.

———. 1994. *The State of the World's Children—1994.* New York: UNICEF.

U.S. Bureau of the Census. 1972. *Statistical Abstract of the United States: 1972* (93rd edition). Washington, D.C.

———. 1975. *Historical Statistics of the United States: Colonial Times to 1970.* Bicentennial Edition, Part 1. Washington D.C.

———. 1985. *Statistical Abstract of the United States: 1986* (106th edition). Washington, D.C.

———. 1986. *Statistical Abstract of the United States: 1987* (107th edition). Washington, D.C.

———. 1991. *Statistical Abstract of the United States: 1990* (111th edition). Washington, D.C.

———. 1993. *Statistical Abstract of the United States: 1993* (113th edition). Washington, D.C.

———. 1994. *Statistical Abstract of the United States: 1994* (114th edition). Washington, D.C.

U.S. National Center for Health Statistics. 1960. *Vital Statistics of the United States: 1960.* Vol. 1. Natality. Washington, D.C.

———. 1978. *Vital Statistics of the United States: 1975.* Vol. 1. Natality. DHEW Publication No.(PHS) 78-1113. Washington, D.C.

Van Gelder, David W. 1978. Report of the President. *AAP News and Comments* 29(3):2–8.

Van Ingen, P. 1921. *The History of Child Welfare Work in the U.S.: A Half Century of Public Health.* New York: American Public Health Association.

Vandersall, Thornton A. 1963. The Disgruntled Pediatrician Syndrome. *Pediatrics* 32(3):465.

Vaughan Victor C., R. James McKay, and Richard E. Behrman, Eds. 1979. *Nelson Textbook of Pediatrics.* Philadelphia: W. B. Saunders.

Veeder, Borden S. 1922. Child Hygiene and the Private Physician. *Journal of the AMA* 79(27):2228–2229.

———. 1923. Pediatrics and the Child. *Journal of the AMA* 81(7):517–518.

———. 1935. Trends of Pediatric Education and Practice. *American Journal of Diseases of Children* 50(1):1–10.

———. 1938. Periods in the Life of the American Pediatric Society: Infancy. *Transactions of the American Pediatric Society* 50:49–55.

———. Ed. 1957. *Pediatric Profiles.* St. Louis: C. V. Mosby.

———. 1958. Pediatric Practice and Its Rewards. *Journal of Pediatrics* 52(6):769–770.

Waserman, Manfred J. 1972. Henry L. Coit and the Certified Milk Movement in the Development of Modern Pediatrics. *Bulletin of the History of Medicine* 46(4):359–390.

Washburn, Alfred H. 1951. Pediatric Potpourri. *Pediatrics* 7(2):299–306.

Webb, E. J., D. T. Campbell, R. D. Schwartz, and L. Sechrest. 1966. *Unobtrusive Measures: Nonreactive Measures in the Social Sciences.* Chicago: Rand-McNally.

Wegman, Myron E. 1994. Annual Statistics of Vital Statistics—1993. *Pediatrics* 94(6):792–803.

Weinberger, Howard L., and Frank A. Oski. 1984. A Survey of Pediatric Resident Training Programs Five years After the Task Force Report. *Pediatrics* 74(4):523–526.

Welch, Henry. 1958. Antibiotics: 1943–1955. Pp. 70–87 in *The Impact of the Antibiotics in Medicine and Society,* edited by Iago Galdston. New York: International Universities Press.

Westoff, Charles F., and Norman B. Ryder. 1977. *The Contraceptive Revolution.* Princeton, N.J.: Princeton University Press.

Weston, Jerry L. 1984. Ambiguities Limit the Role of NPs and PAs. *American Journal of Public Health* 74(1):6–7.

Wheatley, George M. 1961a. Our Specialty—A New Look. *Pediatrics* 27(5):836–837.

———. 1961b. Adolescence. *Pediatrics* 27(1):159–160.

White House Conference on Child Health and Protection. 1932. *Child Health Centers: A Survey.* Report of the Subcommittee on Health Centers. New York: Century.

White, Forrest P. 1965. What Future for the Pediatrician? *Medical Economics* 42(10):120–135.

White, Park Jerauld. 1955. New Pediatricians: New Pediatrics. *Pediatrics* 16(4):537–540.

Willard, William R. Chairman. 1966. *Meeting the Challenge of Family Practice.* Report of the Ad Hoc Committee on Education for Family Practice of the Council of the American Medical Association. Chicago: American Medical Association.

Willard, William R., and C. H. Ruhe. 1978. The Challenge of Family Practice Reconsidered. *Journal of the AMA* 240(5):454–458.

Williams, Cicely D. 1973. Health Services in the Home. *Pediatrics* 52(6):773–781.

Wilson, James L. 1964. Growth and Development of Pediatrics—Presidential Address 1964. *Journal of Pediatrics* 5(6):984–991.

Wineberg, Julius J. 1959. Letter to the Editor. *Pediatrics* 23(5):1007–1008.

Winslow, Charles E. A. 1923. *The Evolution and Significance of the Modern Public Health Campaign.* New Haven, Connecticut: Yale University Press.

Woolgar, Steve, and Dorothy Pawluch. 1985a. Ontological Gerrymandering: The Anatomy of Social Problems Explanations. *Social Problems* 32(3):214–227.

———. 1985b. How Shall We Move Beyond Constructivism. *Social Problems* 33(2):159–162.

Work, Henry H. 1970. Pediatric Globalism. *Pediatrics* 46(2):173–174.

Yancy, W. S. 1975. Behavioral Pediatrics and the Practicing Pediatrician. *Pediatric Clinics of North America* 22(3):685–694.

Yankauer, Alfred, John P. Connelly, and Jacob J. Feldman. 1970. Pediatric Practice in the United States with Special Attention to Allied Health Worker Utilization. *Pediatrics* 45(3):521–551.

Yankauer, Alfred, Sally Tripp, Priscilla Andrews, and John P. Connelly. 1972. The Cost of Training and Income Generation Potential of PNPs. *Pediatrics* 49(6):878–887.

Zack, Brian G. 1981. Adolescent Medicine: Subspecialty or Outcast? *Pediatrics* 68(5):731–733.

Zelizer, Viviana A. 1985. *Pricing the Priceless Child: The Changing Social Value of Children.* New York: Basic Books.

Zietz, Dorothy. 1959. *Child Welfare: Services and Perspectives.* New York: Wiley.

Zola, Irving K. 1972. Medicine as an Institution of Social Control. *Sociological Review* 20:487–504.

Index